Acid Reflux Diet 2020

The Complete Diet Plan for Acid Reflux Disease.
How to Cook Healthy Food for Prevent GERD and
LPR with a 30-Day Meal Plan with Delicious, Quick
& Easy Low-Acid Recipes. Including Gluten Free,
Vegan and Alkaline

Elizabeth Ryan

Copyright © 2020 by Elizabeth Ryan

means or in printed format. Recording of this publication is strictly prohibited and any storage of this document is not allowed unless with written permission from the publisher.

The information provided herein is stated to be truthful and consistent, in that any liability, in terms of inattention or otherwise, by any usage or abuse of any policies, processes, or directions contained within is the solitary and utter responsibility of the recipient reader.

Under no circumstances will any legal responsibility or blame be held against the publisher for any reparation, damages, or monetary loss due to the information herein, either directly or indirectly. Respective authors own all copyrights not held by the publisher.

Contents

ACID REFLUX DIET OR GERD.................................1

    Problems with Conventional Treatments For Acid
Reflux 5

    Advantages and disadvantages 13

    Basic Myths and Questions 15

    Foods to Avoid While on GERD/Acid Reflux Diet...22

    Acid Reflux: Foods to Avoid 26

    Symptoms of Acid Reflux............................28

CITRUS FRUITS AND ACID REFLUX 32

    Tips for Hyperacidic Patients......................33

    Hypoacidic Tips for Patients. 34

    How To Deal with Acid Reflux in General 36

    Other Natural Remedies, Including Supplements and
Essential Oils 37

    Key Points on Acid Reflux Diet and Other Remedies 45

GETTING STARTED WITH THE ACID REFLUX
DIET...47

    Your Calorie and Nutrition Goals 48

    Hydration Tips 49

    Basic food item Staples...............................50

Formula Ideas..53

Preparing and Meal Planning 55

The most effective method to Avoid Acid Reflux.......57

Straightforward remedies for heartburn help..............66

Cooking Your Way to Less Reflux...............75

THE LOW DOWN ON ACID DIET.........................85

HEARTBURN,ACID REFLUX, AND GERD
DURING PREGNANCY...93

Symptoms of indigestion and heartburn....................95

Meds for indigestion and heartburn.........................101

Causes of indigestion in pregnancy..........................103

ACID REFLUX (GERD) IN CHILDREN: CAUSES,
SYMPTOMS, AND TREATMENT 109

Acid Reflux Symptoms In Children..........................109

Appropriate Time To Take Your Child To The
Doctor. 113

Causes Of Acid Reflux In Children 114

Causes Of GERD In Children 115

Treatment For Children Suffering from Acid Reflux
And GERD 119

Characteristic Remedies For Acid Reflux In Children
....122

Foods To Avoid To Prevent Acid Reflux.................127

THE MOST EFFECTIVE METHOD TO TREAT
BAD BREADTH FROM ACID REFLUX.................150

Indications that Acid Reflux Caused Your Bad Breath
.... 153

Bad Breath And Acid Reflux 157

How To Treating Acid Reflux.................................. 160

ACID REFLUX RECIPES 164

Acid reflux formula: Pan burned tilapia................... 165

Acid reflux amicable formula: Asparagus and green
bean serving of mixed greens 168

Acid Reflux Friendly Recipe: Black Bean Burger 171

Banana pecan biscuits.. 174

Slow cooker chicken and grain stew 178

Chicken cutlets with sauteed mushrooms................ 181

Marinated mushroom sandwich............................... 185

Entire wheat pasta serving of mixed greens.............. 186

Asparagus quiche... 187

Banana Ginger Energy Smoothie 191

Function Apple Honeydew Smoothie 192

Muesli-Style Oatmeal.. 193

Moment Polenta With Sesame Seeds 194

Quiet Carrot Salad.. 195

Dark Bean and Cilantro Soup.................................. 196

Chicken and Mushroom Cheese Bake...................... 197

Rich Hummus 199

Watermelon and Ginger Granite.............................. 200

Asparagus quiche......................................201

Banana Ginger Energy Smoothie.............................205

Function Apple Honeydew Smoothie......................206

Muesli-Style Oatmeal..207

Moment Polenta with Sesame Seeds........................208

Quiet Carrot Salad 209

Dark Bean and Cilantro Soup 210

Delightful Cantaloupe Gazpacho 211

Rich Hummus 212

Watermelon and Ginger Granite............................213

Butternut squash soup..214

Broiler steamed tilapia..216

Mustard pork midsection with cauliflower puree.....217

Stuffed mushroom tops...219

Braised short ribs...222

Little lasagna cups 224

Smaller than usual lasagna cups 227

Handcrafted granola parfait....................................230

Enchiladas Verde..231

Pasta primavera with entire wheat pasta..................233

Curry almond chicken...235

Balsamic Chicken Salad...236

Cooked salmon with mango nectar soy coat............239

Chicken tortilla soup..240

Coconut rice pudding...241

Sweet pea smoothie..243

Chicken and Red Potatoes 245

Simple hamburger (or pork) burgundy....................248

Stuffed turkey moves "cordon bleu."......................249

Crisp vegetable and white bean soup.......................252

Prepared chicken and wild rice...............................253

Vegetable macaroni and cheddar.............................254

Small spinach serving of mixed greens.....................255

Barbecued Caesar swordfish 256

Lentil burgers...257

Hawaiian-style ahi sandwich with coconut slaw.......260

Chicken pot pie 261

Banana date mousse..264

Salmon burgers with carrot slaw and miso yogurt....265

Smooth split pea soup...269

Great morning natural product plate of mixed greens
....272

Sound jumble plate of mixed greens........................273

Carrot milkshake smoothie 274

Raisin walnut and carrot bread................................275

Exquisite Dover sole...276

Peachy shoemaker 277

Outing potato serving of mixed greens 280

Excursion potato plate of mixed greens.....................281

Meat and mushroom skillet......................................282

Prepared French fries...285

Outlandish Asian rice..288

Home-style southern bread rolls...............................289

Heated bananas...290

Twice heated potatoes..291

Frosty mango smoothie..292

Carolina potato pie..293

Apple smoothie with wheat germ............................294

Structure your own' breakfast granola.....................296

Natively constructed turkey soup............................299

White Fish Veronica...300

Vegetarian chia burger...301

ACID REFLUX DIET OR GERD

What Is Acid Reflux?

Acid reflux, additionally called heartburn, is brought about by acidic digestive juices crawling up from the stomach and entering over into the throat. It is identified with gastroesophageal reflux disease (or GERD), the more serious type of these problems. Acid reflux causes a consuming sensation, practically like your chest or throat "is one fire."

A great many people expect that eating foods high in acid and delivering a lot of stomach acid causes heartburn/GERD symptoms. The inverse is, by all accounts genuine. These problems won't be relieved medium-term with dietary changes or different alterations. However, you can discover huge help reasonably soon on the off chance that you stay with a more beneficial method for living.

Around 4–10 percent of all grown-ups experience symptoms run of the mill of acid reflux or GERD every day, and week after week for up to 30 percent of those living in Western nations! Since we're all unique, it's fundamental to discover the mix of acid reflux conventions portrayed underneath that is best for you. Indeed, progressing research is concentrating not simply on pharmaceutical medications for the alleviation of acid reflux, yet in addition to way of life alterations. For instance, a few changes you might need to attempt to incorporate eating an acid reflux diet, needle therapy, yoga, work out, weight reduction, and elective treatments.

Acid Reflux Symptoms, Causes and Risk Factors

For the vast majority with acid reflux or heartburn, symptoms include:

- ❖ Chest agonies and consuming sensations
- ❖ Bitter taste in your mouth

- ❖ Trouble resting, including awakening feeling like you're stifling or hacking in the night
- ❖ Dry mouth
- ❖ Gum aggravation, including delicacy and dying
- ❖ Bad breath
- ❖ Gas, burping, and stomach swelling after suppers.
- ❖ Sometimes queasiness and loss of craving.
- ❖ And a huge number of different symptoms relying upon how seriously the throat gets kindled or harmed.

GERD symptoms are like acid reflux symptoms, albeit here and there progressively serious. The basic explanation that acid reflux/heartburn creates is because of the brokenness of the lower esophageal sphincter (LES). Generally, the LES "keeps a top of things" by keeping acid from streaming back up through the throat. (3) While the stomach has a worked in a coating that shields it from feeling "consumed" because of the nearness of acid, the throat doesn't. Since it's not protected like the stomach is, the throat can begin to disintegrate and create difficulties after some time when acid reflux isn't dealt with. Thus, tissue scarring and even arrangement of malignant esophageal growth in extreme cases may happen.

While individuals build up this digestive issue for various reasons, causes of acid reflux that add to difficult symptoms for some individuals include: Eating foods excessively quick, without biting appropriately, or setting aside an effort to process. Indeed, in our quick-paced society, this is accepted to be one of the most widely recognized causes of infrequent acid reflux/heartburn.

- ❖ Overeating, which assesses the digestive framework and adds strain to the stomach
- ❖ Eating just 1-2 major suppers for every day, as opposed to dividing dinners out.
- ❖ Obesity and being overweight
- ❖ Older age, which influences an acid generation

- ❖ History of Hiatal hernias
- ❖ Pregnancy
- ❖ Consuming certain foods that will, in general, irritate the digestive framework, including handled foods, sugary tidbits, refined oils, fried foods, and prepared meats.
- ❖ Taking certain physician recommended prescriptions, including rehash anti-infection agents or those used to treat hypertension, asthma, joint inflammation, heart problems, and osteoporosis.
- ❖ High measures of ceaseless pressure
- ❖ Deficiencies in specific supplements
- ❖ Smoking, liquor, and high caffeine use

Problems with Conventional Treatments For Acid Reflux

Acid reflux, heartburn, and GERD are normally treated with prescriptions or over-the-counter medications to bring down agony. At times these are utilized when symptoms are starting to erupt, while in different cases, they are taken day by day to avoid symptoms.

The three principal sorts of medications to treat acid reflux symptoms or those brought about by GERD are: antacids, H2RAs , and PPIs (proton siphon inhibitors). Previously, you may have taken a portion of these items and pills to determine your symptoms.

Acid reflux or GERD drugs have been found to add to symptoms like poor digestion, bad-tempered inside disorder (IBS), melancholy, paleness, and exhaustion. Long haul utilization of gastric acid concealment, similar to proton siphon inhibitors (PPIs) or antacid meds, are even connected with an expanded risk of C. difficile infections. Subsequently, major problems that can create incorporate loose bowels aroused digestive organs and draining ulcers. Patients who are at the most serious risk for reactions from PPIs incorporate the old, those with certain incessant ailments, and those taking expansive range anti-infection agents.

The FDA has cautioned patients consuming these medications that they ought to quickly contact their medicinal services proficient and look for care on the off chance that they create looseness of the bowels that don't improve.

What is the Acid Reflux Diet?

The acid reflux diet is intended to help improve digestive wellbeing, dispose of the symptoms of acid reflux, and lift your insusceptible framework to avoid this kind of stomach issue. The measure of acid your stomach produces is, to a great extent, subject to the foods that you eat, so forming your diet to avoid acid-delivering foods is basic. The more typical name for acid reflux is heartburn, a condition where digestive juices enter the throat, which can bring about a consuming sensation. A portion of the other regular symptoms of acid reflux incorporate chest agonies and issue certain processing foods. This diet can re-set your stomach and additionally build up sound dietary propensities, which will anticipate these symptoms later on.

The acid reflux diet is an eating plan intended for individuals who experience the ill effects of acid reflux to keep symptoms under control. Acid reflux happens when stomach acid washes back up from your stomach into your throat, causing symptoms like heartburn, a snugness in your chest, or a severe preference for your mouth.

At the point when acid reflux is constant, it's known as gastroesophageal reflux disease (GERD). The acid reflux diet means to monitor GERD by avoiding trigger foods. This diet isn't perfect for everybody, except numerous who battle with acid reflux discovers help from awkward symptoms.

The acid reflux diet is an eating plan intended for individuals who experience the ill effects of acid reflux to keep symptoms under control. Acid reflux happens when stomach acid washes back up from your stomach into your throat, causing symptoms like heartburn, a snugness in your chest, or a harsh preference for your mouth.

At the point when acid reflux is incessant, it's known as gastroesophageal reflux disease (GERD). The acid reflux diet plans to monitor GERD by avoiding trigger foods. This diet isn't perfect for everybody, except numerous who battle with acid reflux discovers help from awkward symptoms.

The acid reflux diet limits foods that can intensify symptoms of reflux. Specialists concur that nourishment, and another way of life factors, can majorly affect symptoms. It's useful to work with a specialist when constraining foods to guarantee supplement parity and fulfillment are kept up.

Foundation

The acid reflux diet was planned as an approach to battle acid reflux, a condition that happens when stomach acid streams again into the throat. The diet is regularly prescribed by specialists to anticipate and treat a huge number of unwanted symptoms, including:

- ❖ Frequent burping or hiccuping
- ❖ Chronic swelling or indigestion
- ❖ A consuming sensation in your throat
- ❖ A harsh preference for your mouth
- ❖ Tightness or distress in your chest
- ❖ Heartburn
- ❖ Difficulty gulping

Ceaseless acid reflux can transform into GERD, which is a genuine ailment that can prompt different difficulties whenever left untreated.

Given restricted research and narrative proof of patients, wellbeing experts have arrived at the resolution that a few foods may trigger acid reflux and the acid reflux diet plans to avoid those foods.

Research has discovered the relationship between acid reflux and elevated cholesterol foods, fatty and fried foods, citrus fruits, acidic foods, caffeine, spicy foods, dairy, and carbonated drinks. This way, the acid reflux diet urges individuals to confine those foods.

How It Works

There's nobody acid reflux diet that suits everybody. While there is a general enemy of reflux rules to pursue, what works best is exceptionally individualized. For instance, some discover chocolate triggers reflux, yet on the off chance that you can eat chocolate with no distress, don't hesitate to continue getting a charge out of it.

Furthermore, way of life factors influence acid reflux—you should represent things like tobacco use, stress, work out, rest designs, dietary patterns (e.g., huge late-night suppers), and liquor utilization, notwithstanding your diet.

If you figure you would profit by following the acid reflux diet, work with a doctor or enlisted dietitian who can assist you with finding your trigger foods, like an end diet for nourishment sesitivities.

When you discover your triggers, you'll need to avoid them. Most wellbeing experts likewise prescribe that eating littler suppers, all the more now and again, for the day to battle acid reflux.

Practically every examination study done on GERD and acid reflux focuses on a poor, prepared diet as a contributing component. What's more, it's anything but difficult to indulge handled foods and in the process of disregarding careful eating rehearses. While everybody's gut is extraordinary and we as a whole respond to different foods in our very own special way, there are normal nourishment sensitivities that appear to trigger acid reflux in numerous individuals. Make certain to concentrate on removing these "recurrent guilty parties" from your diet first.

For good digestive wellbeing and help from torment, it's imperative to choose natural foods free from

GMOs as regularly as could be allowed. Expanding fiber admission, supporting solid microbes with probiotic-rich foods and enhancements, lessening grains, and eating excellent protein will likewise help ensure the digestive tract. Also, these progressions to your diet diminish risk factors like aggravation, heftiness, and inconveniences attached to genuine interminable diseases.

Advantages and disadvantages

Following the acid reflux diet may assist you with pinpointing trigger foods and along these lines avoid acid reflux. Furthermore, this diet may likewise assist you with fitting more vegetables, lean protein, and entire grains into your diet while restricting undesirable fats and fried nourishment included sugar and pop.

There are likewise therapeutic medicines, for example, various pills or medical procedures, to treat interminable acid reflux, yet changing your diet is an extraordinary spot to begin—also, it's simpler and more moderate than a solution or a methodology.

You may be amazed to discover that notwithstanding a solid sponsorship, there's, in reality, almost no proof that a trigger-based diet (or any diet whatsoever) is successful for treating GERD. The American College of Gastroenterology doesn't suggest this methodology because the association isn't clear. Besides, end diets can be hard to pursue for the initial not many weeks, and you may have withdrawal symptoms in case you're accustomed to eating sugar and drinking espresso day by day.

Advantages and disadvantages thought of you as may, in any case, have karma with the acid reflux diet. Simply counsel with an expert before starting.

Basic Myths and Questions

On the off chance that you have acid reflux or GERD, you may have a couple of inquiries concerning the acid reflux diet.

Will changing my diet alone dispose of my symptoms?

Likely not. Acid reflux can happen from an assortment of individual components or a mix of elements. You may need to make the way of life changes that include: stopping tobacco use, starting an activity plan, getting more rest, diminishing pressure, diminishing liquor utilization, shedding pounds, and modifying your eating designs.

Wouldn't I be able to do a normal end diet simply?

No. A customary disposal diet tries to find nourishment hypersensitivities or sensitivities. It works by removing the entirety of the significant allergens: soy, eggs, tree nuts, dairy, gluten, fish, caffeine, sugar, and liquor. While a portion of those foods covers with the rebellious acid reflux foods, the diets have various objectives.

Does the acid reflux diet work for everybody?

While it is conceivably viable, everybody's trigger foods are unique, and a few people may not discover accomplishment with the acid reflux diet. Also, as referenced prior, it's not simply dieting that adds to acid reflux.

There's very confirmation that the acid reflux diet works for anybody—the diet depends on restricted proof between singular foods or mixes and acid reflux symptoms, for example, cholesterol.

How It Compares

Even though the acid reflux diet is intended to meet a specific objective, it's as yet like some other well-known diets. Think about these brisk correlations:

Disposal diet

- ❖ A trigger-nourishment diet that means to reveal nourishment hypersensitivities or sensitivities
- ❖ Very prohibitive in initial not many weeks—removes all known significant allergens.

Mediterranean diet

- ❖ A well-inquired about good dieting arrangement that emulates the style of eating found in Mediterranean nations
- ❖ Focuses on fruits, vegetables, solid fats, entire grains, and lean protein
- ❖ Not prohibitive
- ❖ Can be pursued without one-on-one direction from a wellbeing proficient

Run Diet

- ❖ A well-regarded and vigorously inquired about eating plan to bring down circulatory strain, or hypertension.
- ❖ Very adjusted and centers around the utilization of entire, supplement thick foods.

- ❖ Heavy center around salt admission
- ❖ Can be pursued without one-on-one direction from a wellbeing proficient

Beginning

In case you're prepared to begin on the acid reflux diet, discover a pen and a bit of paper. Start by making a considerable number of foods that you think may trigger your symptoms. At the point when you're prepared to begin, cut out those foods—simply ensure you have substitution thoughts while you're in this end-stage.

Disposal diets are done best with the assistance of an expert, who can tell you when to include foods back in and in what request. It is useful to keep a nourishment journal and take notes on your symptoms: Do they reduce in force? Recurrence? Do they leave inside and out? More often than not, in the reintroduction stage, foods are included back each in turn, with a few days between foods.

While picking a diet, it's imperative to pick one that will assist you with arriving at your objectives.If you will likely decrease or kill your acid reflux symptoms, at that point, the acid reflux diet may merit going after for you. Remember that the acid reflux diet is progressively similar to a lot of harsh rules as opposed to an exacting eating plan. Flex it to address your issues, and counsel with a wellbeing proficient for direction. If the diet doesn't help, it might be a great opportunity to think about other treatment alternatives.

Listed are the foods that can improve acid reflux and treat GERD:

- ❖ Kefir and yogurt help balance sound microscopic organisms in the stomach, supporting digestion and alleviating the digestive tract. Select items that have live and dynamic societies that have been aged for 24 hours.

- ❖ Bone soup produced using grass-bolstered meat, slow-cooked to remove fundamental mixes including collagen, glutamine, proline, and glycine.
- ❖ Fermented vegetables, including kimchi and sauerkraut.
- ❖ Kombucha pressed with sound microscopic organisms and probiotics.
- ❖ Apple juice vinegar adjusts stomach acid and decreases the symptoms of acid reflux. Blend one tablespoon of crude apple juice vinegar with some water and drink five minutes before eating.
- ❖ Coconut water and high content of potassium and electrolytes that help to keep the body hydrated. Taste coconut water for the day and drink a glass before bed to help keep acid reflux under control. Coconut water can likewise be made into kefir, which includes extra sound probiotics into the stomach that people with acid reflux urgently need.
- ❖ Attempt to devour one tablespoon of coconut oil every day. For instance, spread it on grew

grain bread or consolidated into different foods. The lauric acid and other regular mixes help to battle aggravation, to support invulnerability, and to slaughter candida.

- ❖ Green verdant vegetables
- ❖ Artichokes
- ❖ Asparagus
- ❖ Cucumbers
- ❖ Pumpkin and other squash
- ❖ Wild-got fish and salmon
- ❖ Healthy fats including coconut oil and ghee
- ❖ Raw bovine's milk cheddar
- ❖ Almonds
- ❖ Honey

A considerable lot of these foods are remembered for The GAPS diet, a dietary arrangement I suggest for individuals with digestive problems that spotlights on entire foods. The GAPS diet can be useful for treating conditions like IBS, cracked gut, ADHD, and numerous different conditions too close to acid reflux. Indeed, GAPS is a diet wealthy in new natural vegetables, unfenced chicken and grass-nourished meat, and bone stock. It likewise fuses sound herbs or plants, for example, aloe vera, parsley, ginger, and fennel, which can alleviate the digestive tract. (8)

Foods to Avoid While on GERD/Acid Reflux Diet

Specific foods are recognized to be the cause of acid reflux symptoms. This foods are said to "fan the flares" of acid reflux, incorporate substantial foods, cheap food, prepared cheeses, chocolate, liquor, and caffeine.

Here are foods to avoid that normally exacerbate acid reflux symptoms:

❖ Alcohol. While a few people feel OK having modest quantities of liquor with some restraint, others discover brew, alcohol, and wine to be a portion of the more regrettable offenders. Expend modest quantities one after another alongside a lot of water to test how you respond. Additionally, it avoids liquor near sleep time, or when eating different foods that can trigger symptoms.

❖ Caffeine. Drinks like espresso, tea, and caffeinated drinks can aggravate a kindled throat and modify how the sphincter functions.

❖ Carbonated drinks. This incorporates sodas, liquor, caffeinated drinks, even seltzer or shimmering water, and so on.

❖ Sugar and fake sugars. Both are the reason for irritation much of the time and can prompt over-eating, quick eating, and weight gain.

❖ Fried foods. Fatty foods will, in general, sit in the stomach for quite a while and are difficult to process appropriately. Subsequently, this can trigger the surplus acid generation.

❖ Processed foods made with bunches of salt, corn, and potato. These incorporate chips, wafers, grains, and so on. An exceptionally high level of bundled items are made with some sort of prepared corn fixing, so read fixing names and attempt to expend increasingly natural "entire foods." An excess of sodium is another large issue that is connected to the utilization of bundled items. One Swedish investigation that pursued in excess of 1,000 individuals found that the individuals who devoured a high-sodium diet have essentially higher paces of acid reflux.

❖ Chocolate. Numerous individuals locate that removing cocoa/chocolate from their diet improves symptoms. Considering numerous chocolate items contain prepared, fats, caffeine, and sugar (a "triple whammy"), it's one of the most exceedingly terrible guilty parties.

❖ Dairy items. Little out of every odd individual has a negative response to dairy foods, similar to yogurt or cheddar, yet some do. Milk items contain calcium, sugar, and normal fat, which would all be able to trigger the arrival of increasingly acid from the stomach.

❖ Vegetable oils, including canola oil. Prepared oils, like fried and fatty foods, are found in bunches of bundled bites that can trigger irritation.

❖ Spicy foods. Flavors like cayenne, bean stew, cinnamon, or pepper are different sorts of fixings that can be commonly solid. In any case, spicy foods are known to exacerbate the consuming sensation related to acid reflux in certain patients. Since flavors influence everybody unexpectedly, test your very own symptoms to perceive how you feel while devouring them. Rather, blander foods made with less zest may be a superior choice if your symptoms deteriorate.

❖ Tomatoes, tomato items, and onions. Even though they are solid all in all, these vegetables can trigger symptoms in specific individuals, particularly when eaten in huge sums, (for example, bunches of tomato sauce).

❖ Citrus fruits and squeezes. Citrus fruits are, to some degree, high in acid and exacerbate symptoms.

❖ Creamy/slick arranged to serve of mixed greens dressings.

❖ Mint and peppermint. Mint items appear to aggravate symptoms since they lower pressure in the esophageal sphincter, enabling acid to rise.

❖ Processed grains.

Acid Reflux: Foods to Avoid

Acid reflux suggests the progression of the acidic substance of the stomach into the throat (nourishment pipe), and even the throat and mouth. This prompts heartburn and GERD. The present article gives a rundown of foods to be avoided to avert or control this condition.

Should Citrus Fruits be Avoided?

It is a typical confusion that hyperacidity is the main explanation for acid reflux and that acidic foods should consistently be avoided. Numerous cases, including acid reflux, are brought about by a diminished generation of gastric acid (hypoacidity). Thus, etiology is the main factor in whether citrus fruits ought to be avoided.

Acid reflux is a condition whereby the acidic gastric juices stream from the stomach into the throat, which isn't outfitted to manage acidic conditions. Therefore one encounters heartburn and a harsh taste of the spewed acidic substance.

The retrogressive progression of gastric juices is ordinarily repressed by a roundabout muscle called lower esophageal sphincter (LES), present at the interfacing point among the throat and stomach. This structure capacities like a single direction valve and enables the nourishment bolus to enter the stomach, however, confines the progression of gastric substance into the throat.

Breakdown of LES because of hyperacidity, hypoacidity, unfriendly impacts of drugs, and so on., brings about successive unwinding of this muscle, which prompts acid reflux. This condition may advance to its serious state called gastroesophageal reflux disease (GERD). Visit or nonstop presentation to such acidic substance prompts aggravation of the esophageal tissue, and may likewise prompt erosive esophagitis (irritation of the throat).

Symptoms of Acid Reflux

Heartburn, a consuming sensation in the chest, is the most widely recognized indication related to acid reflux. Other intermittent symptoms experienced include:

- ❖ Burning sensation in the throat
- ❖ Sour preference for mouth
- ❖ Abdominal inconvenience
- ❖ Difficulty and torment while relaxing
- ❖ Difficulty and agony while gulping (dysphagia)
- ❖ Insomnia

Visit scenes, including any of these symptoms, may show the beginning of GERD, and demand proficient restorative guidance.

Foods to Avoid

Basic dietary changes can decrease the symptoms and distress experienced because of acid reflux. Foods to avoid or ease these symptoms, for the most part, incorporate those that are anything but difficult to process and low in fat substance. Despite what might be expected, foods that can disturb or instigate acid reflux incorporate fried foods, high-fat dairy items, pastries, spicy foods, mixed drinks, and so on.

Given beneath is a rundown of foods that must be avoided, or devoured with some restraint while encountering acid reflux:

- ❖ Salted chips
- ❖ French fries
- ❖ Donuts
- ❖ Chocolates
- ❖ Cheese
- ❖ Butter treats
- ❖ Brownies
- ❖ Tabasco sauce

- ❖ Spearmint
- ❖ Chilies
- ❖ Pepper
- ❖ Garlic
- ❖ Onions
- ❖ Tomatoes
- ❖ Ground hamburger
- ❖ Deep-fried meat
- ❖ Processed wieners
- ❖ Marbled sirloin
- ❖ Wine
- ❖ Liquor
- ❖ Tea
- ❖ Coffee
- ❖ Milkshakes
- ❖ Carbonated drinks

Fried foods and high-fat nourishment things are hard to process and are held in the stomach for a more drawn out time. This builds the weight inside the stomach, which actuates acid reflux. Such nourishment things and mixed refreshments debilitate/harm the LES prompting a disappointment in limiting gastric acids to the stomach. Spicy foods disturb the esophageal covering, in this way, expanding the consuming sensation experienced in the throat and chest. They may not instigate acid reflux, yet may disturb the symptoms, and are best avoided.

CITRUS FRUITS AND ACID REFLUX

Strikingly, two unmistakably inverse conditions - hyperacidity (acid dyspepsia) and hypoacidity - can prompt acid reflux. Subsequently, we usually run over grumblings concerning acid reflux deteriorating, regardless of acid concealment treatment and non-extravagance in acidic foods.

Diminished acid generation decreases the effectiveness of digestion, where the chyme is held in the stomach for a more extended period. This presses the LES, and the gastric substance ascends in the throat, causing heartburn. An acid concealment treatment will additionally exasperate the issue and accomplish more damage than anything else.

In this way, people with hyperacidity are encouraged to avoid lime, lemon, oranges, vinegar, and comparable nourishment things with a high acidic substance. In the contradicting condition, those with hypoacidity are educated to expand the admission regarding such foods, to help digestion and reduce acid reflux.

Tips for Hyperacidic Patients

❖ Avoid foods from the rundown of foods that irritate acid reflux (or eat with some restraint), while controlling part consumption.

❖ Juice assortments of acidic nourishment ought to likewise be avoided.

❖ Spicy nourishment ought to be avoided until the condition dies down, where poise ought to be practiced from thereon.

❖ Foods that reason fart, as circulated through drinks and its sort, ought to be gradually dispensed with from your diet.

❖ Maintain an exacting rest timetable of at any rate 7-8 hours every night.

❖ Food segments ought to be little and eaten at various occasions of the day, and not at the same time as a major aspect of an enormous dinner.

❖ Cancel out the utilization of liquor, and point of confinement the number of cigarettes you smoke in a day.

❖ Try to fuse a solid way of life by rehearsing contemplation, pursuing a yoga class, or enjoying light yet strenuous exercise.

❖ Do not starve yourself; in any event, fasting shouldn't be a piece of your daily dietary schedule.

Hypoacidic Tips for Patients.

❖ Get plant sources that can help with hypoacidity such as archangelica, orange strip and the likes.

❖ Include carminatives as a component of your diet; these incorporate caraway, peppermint (avoid if you have an instance of stomach lining aggravation or ulcers), heavenly basil, catnip, and fennel.

- ❖ Consult your PCP for these shifted diet proposals that can help mitigate hypoactivity, just as ask around four treatment choices that could help - prebiotics, probiotics, supplements, and tinctures.

- ❖ Exercise is significant, where it must qualify as thorough and physically burdening.

- ❖ Indulge in spa customs, outings to a loosening up goal, or a quieting action, since stress is a central point of acidic afflictions.

- ❖ Don't enable companions or family to entice you with nourishment decisions that aren't pleasant for your condition. The breaking points your admission of foods that could upset your framework's capacity to deliver acid, and counsel your primary care physician on which foods can be eaten normally, and which ones must be avoided or eaten with some restraint.

It is fundamental to understand the precise reason behind heartburn and stomach distress. This can be dictated by monitoring which foods you expend and watching their belongings after some time. In extreme cases, an expert discussion is a perfect method for managing this, rather than exploring different avenues regarding your wellbeing.

How To Deal with Acid Reflux in General

✓ 'Nourishment triggers' for acid reflux may fluctuate, starting with one individual then onto the next. The ideal approach to make sense of your rundown of 'foods to avoid' is to keep up a nourishment journal and scribble down the foods that messed digestive up.

✓ Sleep on your back, and guarantee that the head is marginally raised.

✗ Refrain from heading to sleep following supper. Go for a walk, read a most loved book, or immerse yourself in a pastime.

The basic way of life changes like normal exercise, utilization of well-adjusted dinners, and a mindful endeavor to avoid dangerous foods is the way to manage acid reflux, just as the physical and mental uneasiness related.

Other Natural Remedies, Including Supplements and Essential Oils

1. Enhancements for Acid Reflux Symptoms:

Notwithstanding eating a sound diet of foods that help to alleviate the symptoms of acid reflux and GERD, it's imperative to add normal enhancements to your diet.

❖ Digestive Enzymes. Take a couple of containers of an excellent digestive catalyst toward the beginning of every supper. They help   foods   completely   review,   and supplements retain appropriately.

❖ Probiotics. Take 25–50 billion units of top-notch probiotics day by day. Adding sound microorganisms adjusts the digestive tracts and group out terrible microscopic organisms that can prompt indigestion, broken gut, and poor assimilation of supplements.

❖ HCL with Pepsin. Take one 650 milligram pill preceding every supper. Add extra pills as important to keep awkward symptoms under control.

❖ Chamomile tea. Taste one cup of chamomile tea preceding bed improved with crude nectar. Chamomile tea diminishes irritation in the digestive tract, supporting sound working.

❖ Ginger tea. Heat a one-inch bit of crisp ginger in 10 ounces of water for 10 minutes. Improve with nectar and taste after dinners or preceding bed. Ginger is utilized for digestive help the world over. If you don't have new ginger on hand, a great ginger enhancement in container structure taken at the beginning of symptoms can help calm symptoms.

❖ Papaya leaf tea. Papain, a catalyst in papaya, helps in digestion by separating proteins. On the off chance that new natural, non-GMO papaya isn't accessible, a natural papaya leaf tea is a decent other option. Eat one cup of new papaya at the beginning of acid reflux symptoms or taste some preceding tea bed.

❖ Magnesium complex enhancement. Take 400 milligrams of a top-notch magnesium supplement two times a day. As referenced above, being lacking in magnesium can cause inappropriate sphincter working, coming about in GERD symptoms. Magnesium is demonstrated to be compelling at treating heartburn.

❖ L-Glutamine. Take five grams of glutamine powder two times every day with suppers. Various research thinks about the show that it recuperates cracked gut and advantages both ulcerative colitis and IBS.

❖ Melatonin. Take six milligrams each night. Research demonstrates that melatonin levels in people with acid reflux are altogether lower than people without acid reflux. Roughly 50 percent of people that take melatonin for 12 weeks had symptoms improve or leave. (12)

2. Fundamental Oils

Lemon and lemon fundamental oil can be useful for controlling acid reflux in certain patients, even though not every person reacts to this similarly (some make some hard memories with citrus items, in any event at first). You can have a go at expending lemon squeeze alongside a cut of new ginger in your water every day. You can likewise include a drop or two of lemon basic oil to water, or spot one drop of remedial evaluation (unadulterated oil) on your tongue, washing, and gulping.

3. Change The Way You Eat and Chew

❖ Don't gorge eat littler dinners to enable foods to process appropriately. Huge suppers and gorging put additional weight on the sphincter, which thus can bring about spewing forth of acid and unprocessed foods.

❖ Don't devour nourishment three hours before bed—enable your stomach to process the foods from the supper and taste a natural tea with nectar to calm digestive miracle.

❖ Chew foods completely—the vast majority today don't bite their nourishment enough; recall, digestion begins in the mouth! Since the more you separate foods preceding gulping, the simpler time your stomach will have processing them.

❖ Wear open to attire in the wake of eating—avoid tight-fitting dress and belts, particularly during supper time. These can make symptoms, weight, and torment more awful.

4. Other Lifestyle Changes and Tips

Restoring acid reflux and GERD requires a multi-prong approach. Way of life changes like eating a sound diet, avoiding nourishment triggers, and taking the correct enhancements can all truly help. Furthermore, a high level of sufferers will discover help from rolling out different improvements to how and when they eat, alongside how they rest and move their bodies.

Here are tips that can lessen the beginning of acid reflux symptoms by diminishing normal triggers:

❖ Sleep on your side and raise your head. Attempt to lift the leader of your bed 4–6 inches, since laying absolutely level down in bed may aggravate symptoms. Use squares to raise the bed, not simply cushions. This is superior to anything simply propping up your head with pads, which can mess neck up. Raising your head around evening time can help keep acid in the stomach and mitigate symptoms of acid reflux and GERD. Accordingly, there is a continuous research study testing rest positions and their impact on acid reflux symptoms around evening time.

❖ Don't twist around. Twisting around from the midriff to assuage torment will probably not help. Indeed, twisting around may even aggravate symptoms by pressing the stomach.

❖ Manage stress. Stress exacerbates symptoms of acid reflux by expanding acid creation in the stomach. It's critical to begin fusing unwinding procedures into your day by day schedule. For instance, attempt yoga, reflection, craftsmanship treatment, or whatever encourages you to oversee pressure adequately.

❖ Acupressure. Certain reflex focuses at the base of the rib confine are related to digestion and can help assuage the symptoms.

❖ Don't depend on drugs. As referenced above, the physician recommended meds just incidentally treat the symptoms. For long haul help, you should change your diet and way of life. If you are going to consume medications for torment, take them near sleep time for the most alleviation.

❖ Exercise. Exercise modestly. Indeed, contemplates show that thorough exercise and running can foment the digestive tract and cause acid reflux. Exercise prior in the day.

❖ Smoking. If you smoke, stop as quickly as time permits! Smoking can loosen up your sphincter and cause acid to rise. Recycled smoke can, likewise, exacerbate symptoms.

Precautions When Treating Acid Reflux

Because acid reflux is normal, it doesn't mean it's "typical." If your acid reflux symptoms meddle with your way of life or everyday action, influence your hunger or supplement admission and keep going for over about fourteen days. At that point, think about visiting a specialist. Different motivations to hear an expert point of view on treatment choices incorporate encountering: raspiness, declining of asthma after meals, the torment that is persevering when resting, torment following activity, trouble breathing that happens fundamentally around evening time, looseness of the bowels, and issue gulping for more than one to two days.

Key Points on Acid Reflux Diet and Other Remedies

❖ Acid reflux is brought about by stomach acid crawling up into the throat. Symptoms of acid reflux typically include chest torments, heartburn, an awful preference for the mouth, swelling, gassiness, and trouble processing and gulping appropriately.

❖ Commonand general causes of acid reflux and GERD include: eating a horrible eating routine, over-eating and eating rapidly, pregnancy, history of Hiatal hernias, heftiness, more established age, and unevenness of stomach acid.

5 Natural Remedies for Acid Reflux/GERD

1. Improving your diet
2. Avoiding certain issue foods
3. Reaching a more beneficial weight
4. Taking supportive enhancements
5. Eating littler, progressively adjusted meals

GETTING STARTED WITH THE ACID REFLUX DIET

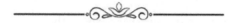

On the acid reflux diet, you'll center on limiting and ideally disposing of symptoms of acid reflux by recognizing trigger foods through an end-stage. For some individuals, trigger foods incorporate high-fat and elevated cholesterol foods, acidic and spicy foods, dairy, espresso, chocolate, and citrus fruits. Everybody has various reactions to various foods, however.

After you distinguish your triggers, you can effectively avoid them and supplant them with solid choices that don't prompt symptoms. Numerous individuals with acid reflux discover accomplishment by eating bunches of vegetables and non-citrus fruits, entire grains, and lean proteins.

Your Calorie and Nutrition Goals

You've presumably seen that most sustenance actualities marks utilize 2,000 calories as an estimation of calorie requirements for the all-inclusive community. They likewise base the level of the prescribed admission for specific supplements off of a 2,000 calorie diet. While 2,000 is a decent broad gauge, everybody's calorie needs differ contingent upon an assortment of components, including:

- ❖ Age
- ❖ Biological sex
- ❖ Height
- ❖ Weight
- ❖ Body creation
- ❖ Activity level
- ❖ Medical conditions

The acid reflux diet doesn't expect you to cling to a particular caloric admission; rather, you'll center on avoiding trigger foods and supplanting them with sound alternatives. To discover what number of calories you need every day, utilize our online calorie adding machine.

Hydration Tips

The familiar aphorism with regards to water admission is "eight glasses every day." But how large are those glasses? Ice or no ice? Such a significant number of inquiries.

In all actuality, there's no all-inclusive perfect number of ounces you should drink every day, much the same as there's no "best" number of calories everybody ought to eat every day. Rather, the aggregate sum of liquid an individual needs to drink is individualized and relies upon an assortment of elements, for example, body weight, activity level, the measure of sweat, to give some examples.

Concerning genuine drink decisions, plain water is normally the best decision with regards to hydration. However, it can get exhausting. You may feel enticed to go after some espresso, pop, or squeeze. However, you won't have any desire to on the acid reflux diet: Caffeine, carbonation, and acidity are key triggers of acid reflux symptoms.

In case you're experiencing difficulty remaining hydrated, have a go at seasoning your water with solidified berries, cut cucumbers, or powdered water flavorings. Hot teas are likewise an incredible method to devour more water; however, you'll need to avoid lemon and mint assortments on the acid reflux diet.

Basic food item Staples

Veggies, veggies, and more veggies. Produce will be the base of your diet when attempting to limit acid reflux symptoms, with moderate parts of lean proteins, non-citrus fruits, and entire grains. You'll avoid fatty, spicy, and acidic foods.

Vegetables: Stock up on verdant greens, root vegetables (sweet potatoes, beets, carrots, and so forth.), and cruciferous vegetables (broccoli, cauliflower).

Fruits: Bananas, pears, apples, coconut, plums, honeydew melon, apricots.

Grains: Choose entire grains like quinoa, bulgur, amaranth, and moved oats.

Protein: Stick to lean proteins without skin, for example, skinless chicken bosoms and 90 percent lean ground turkey.

Agreeable and rebellious foods on the acid reflux diet

In case you're stressed over your meals lacking flavor on the acid reflux diet, expand your points of view with regards to herbs and flavors. Attempt these delightful options in contrast to flavors like cayenne and red pepper that won't cause an agitated in your stomach:

- ❖ Basil
- ❖ Cilantro

- ❖ Rosemary
- ❖ Thyme
- ❖ Oregano

In case you're uncertain about whether a thing is consistent, check the mark for rebellious fixings and sustenance certainties. On the off chance that it's high in fat, sodium, or caffeine, it's likely not agreeable. Consistent things will be insignificantly handled and free of fixings on the rebellious rundown.

Different tips:

Shop the Frozen Section. Solidified fruits and vegetables are similarly as nutritious as new ones, and they keep for more. Solidified produce is typically likewise more affordable than crisp produce.

Purchase Grains in Bulk. You can spare some cash by obtaining moderate dying things in mass, including rice, oats, and different grains.

Purchase Meat When It's on Sale and Freeze it. Getting a lot of proteins is energizing! If you see a two-for-one arrangement at your market, stock up and solidify what you won't use in the following couple of days.

Formula Ideas

When getting started on another diet, you might be overpowered or worried about formula thoughts. On the acid reflux diet, that shouldn't be the situation, as you're permitted to eat an assortment of fulfilling and nutritious foods. Evaluate these formula thoughts for breakfast, lunch, supper, and bite time.

Breakfast

- ❖ Roasted root veggie breakfast tacos
- ❖ Two cuts of entire wheat toast with apricot jelly
- ❖ Healthy entire grain wild blueberry biscuits
- ❖ Warm moved oats with cinnamon, berries, and banana cuts
- ❖ Sweet potato toast with ginger-nectar almond margarine and kiwi cuts

❖ Powdered nutty spread and banana shake

Lunch and Dinner

❖ Tomato sans sauce lasagna

❖ Low-fat chicken parmesan

❖ Grilled vegetable kabobs

❖ Quinoa-stuffed chicken move ups

❖ Spinach plate of mixed greens with strawberries, feta cheddar, and pecans

Bites

❖ Banana with nut spread and cinnamon

❖ Low-fat handcrafted french fries.

❖ Oven-dried persimmon adjusts

❖ Steamed edamame

Treat

❖ Low-fat or nonfat custard, pudding, solidified yogurt, or dessert.

❖ "Nice cream" produced using bananas.

❖ Papaya yogurt and pecan pontoon

❖ Sans fat and breezy heavenly attendant nourishment cupcakes

❖ Low-fat treats

Preparing and Meal Planning

Fortunately, you won't require any unique hardware or extravagant devices to concoct delectable, nutritious meals on the acid reflux diet. These couple of tips can take you far:

Meal Planning and Prepping

You can spare yourself a ton of time, exertion, and cash if you go to the market in light of an arrangement. Before you head out, choose what you need to eat for that week, make a rundown, and stick to it at the store.

After you've arranged your menu and obtained your things, it's an ideal opportunity to cook. The acid reflux diet underscores a lot of foods that can be set up early and heated on the microwave, so you don't need to stress over meals sucking up a lot of your time. Most vegetables, entire grains, and proteins will remain crisp in the cooler for three to five days.

Use What You Have on Hand

If you have a feeling that you're when there's no other option for fixings, you may not be. The acid reflux diet isn't prohibitive, so risks are you can prepare a delectable meal in any event, when you incline that your washroom is getting exposed. Think straightforward, similar to Italian-prepared rice, or moved oats with pounded bananas.

Picking a diet is a major individual choice that requires a lot of consideration over your wellbeing objectives. The acid reflux diet centers around facilitating symptoms of a specific wellbeing condition, and probably won't be most appropriate to individuals who don't have acid reflux. Be that as it may, it's a solid and adjusted diet by and large and doesn't present any perils for the all-inclusive community. I you do have acid reflux, this diet may help and even lead to some auxiliary advantages, similar to weight reduction and more advantageous long haul dietary patterns. Be that as it may, investigate recommends restricting these foods may not generally work, and that trigger foods change from individual to individual.

The most effective method to Avoid Acid Reflux

Beat the consume

While periodic heartburn—which happens when stomach acid sprinkles up into the throat—is upsetting, tenacious acid reflux can be not kidding.

"The acid bites away at the defensive coating of the throat, prompting irritation, ulcer, and obliteration of the covering.

Here are some ways of life changes that can help.

Get in shape

Getting in shape and keeping up a solid body size is perhaps the surest approaches to keep acid reflux under control.

One investigation of more than 10,000 ladies found that even a moderately little increment in weight list could significantly increase the chances of creating gastroesophageal reflux disease (GERD), which is relentless acid reflux.

On the off chance that the normal man or lady sheds 10 pounds, the individual in question will see an improvement in their reflux.

Eat right

Eating inappropriate foods can decline acid reflux, either by expanding the acidic condition of the stomach or by loosening up the lower esophageal sphincter, a valve that goes about as a hindrance between the stomach and the throat.

Fatty foods top the rundown of guilty parties, alongside chocolate, citrus fruits, and squeezes.

In any case, various individuals can respond contrastingly to similar foods. Try to make sense of which foods trouble you the most and avoid them, says Amar Deshpande, MD, collaborator educator of medication at the University of Miami School of Medicine.

Cut back on liquor

Drinking is losing with regards to acid reflux since liquor can expand the stomach's acidity.

Progressively acid methods, it's everything the almost certain it will spill upwards into the throat. Liquor additionally contains various synthetic compounds that can be hard to use and bother the stomach lining.

It's ideal to avoid liquor in case you're inclined to acid reflux.

Cutoff pop

Regular soft drink drinks like Pepsi or Coke contain citrus just as sodium benzoate and different synthetic compounds that can aggravate the gastrointestinal tract. They're ideal to be avoided on the off chance that you have acid reflux.

Carbonated water, then again, shouldn't cause acid reflux.

Try not to smoke

Smoking can cause reflux, not just because it builds acid generation in the stomach, yet additionally because it relaxingly affects the valve between the throat and the stomach.

"That valve regularly remains shut and, when it opens up, it improperly permits acid and stomach substance to come up.

Avoid caffeine

Like smoking, caffeine ups acid creation in the stomach and opens the lower esophageal sphincter.

That implies espresso—even decaffeinated espresso, which still contains modest quantities of caffeine—is off the menu for some individuals with reflux.

Look on the brilliant side. Curtailing the morning cup of Joe may likewise facilitate any butterflies or heart palpitations you've been having.

Check your drugs

Certain prescriptions can raise the risk of acid reflux.

These incorporate bone-reinforcing medications, for example, bisphosphonates, certain circulatory strain drugs, asthma meds containing theophylline, iron and potassium supplements, certain anti-infection agents (antibiotic medication is one), just as headache medicine and ibuprofen, and even fish oil supplements.

Taking a resting pill, for example, Ambien (zolpidem) might be a specific issue. One little investigation found that individuals taking Ambien were bound to have evening time acid reflux and bound to be aroused by it. On the off chance that one drug is giving you inconvenience, converse with your primary care physician about other options, says Dr. Deshpande.

Take a full breath

The correct sort of breathing, similar to the correct sort of nourishment, may likewise ease acid reflux symptoms.

Those in the profound breathing gathering would be advised to personal satisfaction and lower stomach acidity a month and nine months in the wake of beginning the training.

Exercise the correct way

Even though activity is basic for keeping up solid bodyweight, specific sorts of activity may exacerbate acid reflux.

Weight lifting and seat presses, for example, can make additional weight in the midriff, constraining stomach substance up into the throat, says Dr. Deshpande.f

The timing of activity might be a higher priority than the kind of activity, individuals turn out on a vacant stomach. "That will deal with symptoms in most likely 95% of individuals," she says.

Eat little bits

Expending overflowing measures of nourishment at one sitting prompts the stomach to discharge gastrin, a hormone that animates the arrival of stomach acid.

Eating littler sums at increasingly visit interims during the day can be a speedy method to fix—or if nothing else decrease—acid reflux.

Take a stab at eating modest quantities at regular intervals or less for the day.

Try not to eat before sleep time.

Lying level—including when you're dozing or essentially resting to sit in front of the TV or read a book—implies gravity is never again working in support of you.

And that implies stomach acid is bound to go up into your throat instead of remaining down in your stomach.

Rest on an angle

Dozing on a grade can make gravity your companion once more. In any case, ensure your chest—not simply your head—is over your guts. Most of the throat is entirely the chest, not the neck.

Cushions will just lift your head over your chest. A superior thought is to utilize wedge pads or lift the leader of the bed a couple of crawls by utilizing books or a bit of wood under the feet of the bed. One examination found that hoisting the leader of the bed was one of the two best ways of life intercessions to lessen reflux. (The other was getting thinner.)

Get the correct medications.

If way of life mediations aren't working, you should go to any number of over-the-counter and physician endorsed prescriptions, which are accessible for acid reflux.

The three principal classes of medications for this condition are antacids; proton siphon inhibitors (PPIs, for example, Prilosec (omeprazole) or Prevacid (lansoprazole); and histamine 2 (H2) blockers, for example, Pepcid (famotidine) and Zantac (ranitidine).

Be astute about a medical procedure.

Specialists may prescribe the medical procedure for acid reflux. (Medical procedure may likewise help if a hernia is at fault for incessant heartburn.)

A few distinctive insignificantly obtrusive methodologies are accessible, including endoscopic medical procedure and radio ablation (consuming the throat, so it produces scar tissue).

One ongoing examination in the Journal of the American Medical Association found that patients experiencing laparoscopic hostile to reflux medical procedure, which includes fortifying the lower esophageal sphincter with part of the stomach muscle, were similarly prone to be going away five years after the fact as those given standard treatment with the proton siphon inhibitor Nexium (esomeprazole).

Straightforward remedies for heartburn help

- ❖ Ten remedies
- ❖ When to see a specialist
- ❖ Conditions that expansion risk

If you purchase something through a connection on this page, we may procure a little commission, how this functions.

Heartburn is an ailment where the substance of the stomach goes in reverse and upward into the nourishment pipe. Heartburn is otherwise called gastrointestinal reflux.

The stomach and a muscle called the lower esophageal sphincter ordinarily forestall heartburn. In any case, this muscle can, in some cases, unwind and leave the nourishment pipe unprotected from stomach acid.

An individual may encounter heartburn when stomach acid comes into contact with the covering of the nourishment pipe. This can cause the accompanying symptoms:

- ❖ A sentiment of consuming behind the breastbone, neck, and throat
- ❖ Taste changes
- ❖ coughing
- ❖ Voiceraspiness that is aggravated by eating, inclining forward, and resting

The inconvenience of heartburn can keep going for a few hours and may form into a condition called gastroesophageal reflux disease or GERD. GERD can cause visit heartburn, nourishment staying, harm to the nourishment pipe, blood misfortune, and loss of weight.

Ten remedies

Heartburn may advance into a condition called gastroesophageal reflux disease or GERD.

There is a scope of measures individuals can set up to anticipate and treat the symptoms of heartburn. Not all remedies work or are ok for everybody, nonetheless. It is imperative to talk with a specialist about the best solution for you.

Basic remedies for heartburn help incorporate the accompanying:

Smoking discontinuance: Quit smoking and avoiding secondhand smoke.

Adjust dress: Wear baggy garments to avoid pointless weight on the stomach.

Think about physician endorsed meds: People with heartburn ought to likewise talk with their PCP in regards to the utilization of professionally prescribed meds and whether they are directly for the person.

Oversee body weight: People who are overweight or stout may find that diminishing body weight can help. A diet and exercise health improvement plan can lessen symptoms of acid reflux.

Every individual responds to these progressions in an unexpected way, in any case, so it is imperative to talk with a medicinal services supplier before losing a lot of weight.

Raise the leader of the bed: Raising the leader of the bed can enable gravity to decrease heartburn symptoms. Putting obstructs under the top bedposts that raise the bed by somewhere in the range of 6 and 8 inches may work.

Another choice is embeddings froth wedges between the bedding and box spring to raise the edge of the leader of the bed. Cushions are not powerful in lessening heartburn symptoms.

Attempt over-the-counter (OTC) prescriptions: People with heartburn ought to talk with their primary care physician about OTC meds for indication help. A specialist may suggest antacids, acid reducers, including famotidine or ranitidine, or acid blockers, for example, lansoprazole and omeprazole.

Different antacids are accessible to buy on the web.

Utilize homegrown arrangements: The utilization of certain homegrown arrangements may likewise be valuable.

Chamomile is a herb that can lessen symptoms of GERD.

Some prescribed choices for treating the symptoms of GERD include:

- ❖ licorice
- ❖ Slippery elm
- ❖ Chamomile
- ❖ Marshmallow
- ❖ Iberogast, the brand name for a blend of a few herbs that various surveys have demonstrated to be powerful as a GERD treatment

It is significant for individuals to talk with their primary care physician about potential symptoms and medication cooperations before beginning any natural enhancements. Different natural remedies are accessible on the web.

Attempt needle therapy: Although there is restricted proof to help its utilization, needle therapy might be advantageous in soothing the symptoms of heartburn in certain individuals.

Unwind: Stress and strain can cause a wide scope of undesirable reactions, including heartburn. Unwinding strategies, for example, dynamic muscle unwinding, contemplation, or yoga, could give alleviation to certain symptoms.

Roll out some basic improvements to the diet: There are sure dietary triggers that can influence the event and seriousness of heartburn.

Individuals with heartburn ought to avoid the accompanying foods:

- ❖ spicy or oily foods
- ❖ chocolate
- ❖ caffeinated drinks like espresso
- ❖ tomato items
- ❖ garlic
- ❖ peppermint
- ❖ alcohol
- ❖ fizzy drinks

Individuals ought to sit upstanding for at least 3 hours after a meal to lessen heartburn symptoms. Individuals ought to likewise eat littler meals and avoid eating in the 2 to 3 hours before rest.

When to see a specialist

Stopping smoking and avoiding latent smoking can decrease the risk of creating GERD.

Calling a specialist quickly if somebody has any of the accompanying symptoms:

- ❖ Large measures of spewing or regurgitating that are compelling
- ❖ Green, yellow, or bleeding regurgitation, or regurgitation that resembles espresso beans
- ❖ breathing troubles in the wake of regurgitating
- ❖ Mouth or throat torment while eating
- ❖ Painful or troublesome gulping

Conditions that expansion the risk

Pregnancy can expand the risk of GERD.

Variables that expansion the risk of creating GERD include:

- ❖ Pregnancy
- ❖ A hiatal hernia
- ❖ Smoking and inactive smoking
- ❖ Obesity
- ❖ Certain ailments, including dry mouth, asthma, deferred stomach purging, and scleroderma
- ❖ Some prescriptions, for example, those for treating asthma, sensitivities, torment, hypertension, misery, and sleep deprivation
- ❖ Dietary aggravations, including liquor, caffeine, bubbly drinks, chocolate, and acidic foods, and juices

The potential difficulties of heartburn incorporate ulcers, dying, and GERD. Changes to cells in the nourishment funnel may likewise happen, prompting a condition considered Barrett's throat that builds the risk of disease of the nourishment pipe.

Different complexities incorporate nourishment pipe irritation and scope of breathing problems that can include:

- ❖ Asthma
- ❖ Fluid in the lungs
- ❖ coughing
- ❖ A sore throat
- ❖ Hoarseness
- ❖ Pneumonia
- ❖ wheezing

The nourishment channel can likewise be restricted, causing a condition known as an esophageal stricture.

Cooking Your Way to Less Reflux

Cooking Your Way to Less Reflux One way you can assume responsibility for your fight with acid reflux is to start preparing your meals at home. We, as whole expertise simple, it is to simply get a speedy nibble from an eatery after work or between getting the children at school and dropping them off at b-ball practice. Be that as it may, taking the additional effort to get ready meals at home might merit the exertion.

Various foods influence individuals in various manners. Garlic may not trouble you. However, tomato sauce might be your kryptonite. In this way, some portion of the fight will be focusing on what explicit foods trigger your reflux. In the event that you notice you get awful heartburn each time you eat an orange, it's a truly decent sign that you ought to avoid that nourishment. All in all, you ought to avoid foods that contain tomatoes, citrus, chocolate, and mint. Attempt to avoid preparing meals that utilization these specific fixings or make sense of a substitute for the issue fixing.

Another key is attempting to make lighter, lower-fat meals. One simple approach to do this is to prepare or steam your nourishment as opposed to browning or sautéing it. It's a fast and simple approach to cut a portion of the fat from your meal and make it simpler for your body to process. Additionally, take a stab at subbing low-fat yogurt for cream. Little formula changes like that can go far in your battle against reflux. Decreasing your meat parcels and expanding your vegetable servings can likewise be useful. Meats, particularly those high in fat, take more time to exhaust from your stomach, which can be an issue for reflux sufferers. At last, incorporate whatever an entire number of grains in your diet would be prudent (as long as you don't have a hypersensitivity). Entire grains are filling and nutritious.

Drinking water with or directly after your meal can likewise be a decent method to diminish reflux symptoms, particularly heartburn. Water will assist flush with stomaching acid or nourishment out of your throat and withdraw into your stomach. In addition, water can weaken any acid caught in the throat. The more weakened acid is, the less harm it can do. Even though water can be useful, you ought to avoid drinking carbonated water. Carbonated water can expand the weight inside the stomach, which can make the LES glitch.

Similarly, as there are foods you ought to avoid because they can trigger reflux, there are likewise foods that can lessen your risk for reflux. Oatmeal is constantly a decent decision. In addition to the fact that it is sound when all is said in done, but at the same time, it's a low-fat, high-fiber meal that can help mitigate the stomach. Ginger is another extraordinary element for individuals with reflux. It has mitigating characteristics and is frequently used to treat digestive and gastrointestinal issues, for example, reflux. As indicated by certain dietitians, fruits like bananas and melons are frequently endured well by individuals who experience the ill effects of reflux.

In a little level of patients, bananas and melons can exacerbate reflux. By and large, you should search for fruits with a higher pH and avoid acidic fruits like oranges or lemons.

Attempt to join whatever number greens and roots into your diet as could be expected under the circumstances. Vegetables like cauliflower, broccoli, asparagus, and green beans are, for the most part, exceptionally nutritious and won't add to your reflux or GERD, except if you profound fry them. Fennel can be another extraordinary nourishment in the fight against reflux. Studies have indicated that it calms the stomach while improving its capacity and effectiveness. Cut it meager and add it to a plate of mixed greens or a chicken dish for a brisk, solid, sans heartburn meal. And don't fear to eat a couple of complex sugars, for example, dark colored rice. They'll give you fiber and vitality and won't mess up your reflux.

The other thing you'll need to focus on is your decision of protein. Rather than eating high-fat meats, including most red meats, have a go at exchanging over to more slender decisions like chicken or turkey. Now and again, simply changing to a slice of more slender meat can be everything necessary to lessen seething reflux to a sensible condition. The beneficial thing about lean meats is that you can cook them in an assortment of approaches to prevent them from getting exhausted with a similar meal all day every day. Feel free to heat, sear, barbecue, or sauté your poultry, yet make certain to expel the skin since it's high in fat. Additionally, have a go at fusing more fish and fish into your diet. Most sorts of fish are extraordinary low-fat decisions.

Handling Special Situations

A wide assortment of uncommon conditions can impact a treatment plan for acid reflux and GERD. A portion of the more typical gatherings —, for example, pregnant ladies, kids, and the older — are shrouded in Chapter 16. In any case, there are another one of a kind circumstances that can influence your treatment, as well.

One unique case is acid reflux brought about by a hiatal hernia (a condition wherein a little area of the stomach gets pushed up into a gap in the stomach). Littler hernias most likely won't cause numerous recognizable symptoms; in any case, a bigger hernia can cause nourishment and stomach acid to get caught in the throat, causing serious reflux and inconvenience. By and large, specialists may need to do a few systems (for example, an upper endoscopy, esophageal pH test, or esophageal manometry) to check if the hiatal hernia is the reason for the reflux. At the point when your primary care physician has decided the reason, he'll delineate a treatment plan.

There is an assortment of medicines for Hiatal hernias relying upon the particulars of your condition. Now and again, the specialist may endorse over-the-counter antacids or even remedy acid reflux prescription.

Treatment will likewise, for the most part, expect you to alter eating and dozing plans. It'll be significant for you to eat a few little meals daily — attempt to limit the measure of nourishment you eat at any one time. This will help decrease the probability that your reflux or GERD will erupt. You'll additionally need to avoid resting for at any rate of three hours in the wake of eating or drinking. Now and again, your primary care physician will prescribe the medical procedure to address the issue. It's typically a laparoscopic strategy with a recuperation time somewhere in the range of five and ten days.

Treating your reflux or GERD while fighting an ulcer is another uncommon circumstance. For patients with both reflux and ulcers, the agony can be unbearable. Reflux symptoms will, in general, show in the upper chest. However, ulcer torment typically falls between the sternum and navel. If you have a terrible instance of both, you could encounter agony and uneasiness in your entire chest and belly.

On the off chance that your PCP verifies that your ulcer has been brought about by microorganisms living in the mucous covering your stomach (Helicobacter pylori), he'll treat the microscopic organisms with solid antacid meds and anti-infection agents for 7 to 14 days. Fruitful treatment of H. pylori, for the most part, implies that the recuperated stomach lining at that point secretes significantly progressively acid, aggravating your reflux symptoms, at any rate briefly. After the H. pylori have been cleared, you may require a deep-rooted antacid prescription to deal with the reflux.

Indeed, even commonly harmless over-the-counter drugs like headache medicine have been known to cause reflux flare-ups. Different prescriptions that have been routinely connected to reflux and GERD incorporate, anti-toxins, steroids, antihistamines, heart meds, osteoporosis meds, chemotherapy drugs, torment meds, and even potassium and iron enhancements.

Talk straightforwardly with your primary care physician and drug specialist about your reflux symptoms. It's a smart thought to get every one of your meds through a similar drug specialist so she can check for any medication collaborations. The drug specialist may likewise have the option to locate a practically identical prescription that won't affect your reflux. And don't be hesitant to attempt a portion of the standard remedies for reflux, for example, a decent ginger tea or other stomach soothers.

THE LOW DOWN ON ACID DIET

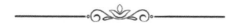

Acid reflux is a surprisingly basic condition that influences a large number of individuals around the world. In the United States, in excess of 50 percent of individuals experience the ill effects of heartburn (one of the essential symptoms of acid reflux). And that is only the infrequent session. Almost 30 percent of Americans experience the ill effects of acid reflux regularly.

Seriousness and recurrence change, essentially starting with one individual then onto the next. You may encounter acid reflux once per month, yet someone else may have reflux day by day and to an incapacitating degree.

For certain individuals, reflux is a long haul issue that they'll need to manage for the remainder of their lives, in spite of making changes. Others find that way of life changes and/or prescription, and the medical procedure can dispense with their symptoms. In any case, heartburn can dramatically affect an individual's life.

Heartburn versus acid reflux When a great many people consider acid reflux, they quickly consider heartburn and utilize the words reciprocally. Despite the fact that reflux and heartburn are connected, they're not something very similar.

Heartburn is, in reality, only a manifestation of acid reflux. Heartburn is an awkward or excruciating consuming sensation in the chest that typically happens after a meal. Exactly the amount it harms shifts from individual to individual, yet additionally from occurrence to case. It can go from a mellow aggravation to an extraordinary, burning agony.

Here's the most effortless approach to recall the distinction among heartburn and acid reflux:

Heartburn is the sensation, while acid reflux is the development or activity that causes the sensation.

The term heartburn can be, to some degree, misdirecting. To start with, heartburn has nothing to do with the heart; it's really identified with the digestive framework, explicitly the throat. Second, heartburn doesn't really consume; it very well may be a general torment or a sentiment of snugness in the chest. Numerous patients have hurried to the emergency clinic, thinking they had a coronary failure, just to discover it was really an intense instance of heartburn. These individuals make some hard memories accepting that an inclination that solid can "simply" be heartburn.

Symptoms of a cardiovascular failure can be unobtrusive from the outset. Try not to attempt to "intense it out." One indication of a coronary episode is chest inconvenience or agony. This may feel like weight, completion, or pressing in your chest. The distress or agony may travel every which way. Different symptoms incorporate body torment, tension, stomach ailment, wooziness, perspiring, and brevity of breath. Main concern: Assume the symptoms you're encountering might be heart-related until a doctor has precluded it.

A great many people will involvement with at least one instance of heartburn in their lifetimes. Fortunate for them, infrequent heartburn ordinarily is nothing to stress over and frequently can be cleared up with an antacid.

If you experience heartburn all the time, you most likely have acid reflux. Much the same as heartburn, acid reflux differs fundamentally in seriousness and recurrence. It very well may be a day by day issue that affects your regular day to day existence, or it tends to be a mellow, incidental disturbance with almost no effect on your exercises.

Extreme, long haul instances of heartburn can prompt analysis of gastroesophageal reflux disease (GERD). The condition is about as charming as the term. Feel free to state it, "GERD." Rhymes with a piece of poop. Typically patients with GERD experience the ill effects of heartburn or other reflux symptoms, in any event, two times per week. If you find that you're experiencing reflux all the time, go to your PCP. Untreated reflux can form into GERD, which can prompt progressively genuine, long haul medical problems.

What acid reflux does Acid reflux be a digestive issue that includes the throat and stomach? At the point when you eat or drink, the substance travel down your throat and into your stomach. At the passage to your stomach is a ring of muscle called the lower esophageal sphincter (LES). The LES is basically a valve for the stomach. It unwinds to enable nourishment or liquid to go into the stomach and then fixes to forestall stomach substance from getting away up the throat.

At the point when you have acid reflux, which generally implies your LES isn't working appropriately. At the point when the LES is working typically, it closes after nourishment or liquid passes. For individuals with acid reflux, this ordinary capacity is forestalled. At times, this is an aftereffect of the muscles being debilitated. In different cases, this is a result of changes in stomach pressure, particularly in the stomach. On different occasions, the LES glitches, and starts opening and shutting itself. Notwithstanding the reason, the breakdown takes into account your stomach substance, including stomach acid, to stream once more into the throat.

The throat is over the stomach, so from a gravitational standpoint, it doesn't appear to be coherent, even with breaking down LES, that anything from the stomach would move back up. This fair goes to show the intensity of what's happening in the stomach. The stomach capacities like a clothes washer — it's amazing. That is the reason you hear, so a lot of clamor on the off chance that you've at any point had your ear close to somebody's stomach after a meal. At the point when you consolidate stirring stomach acid with breaking down LES, somewhat reflux is unavoidable, in spite of gravity.

A manifestation of acid reflux, other than heartburn, is dyspepsia (stomach distress, for the most of the upper guts). Heartburn can likewise make a sentiment of totality or swelling, burping, and sickness, as a rule in the wake of eating. This can prompt spewing forth, which is another normal acid reflux side effect. Spewing forth happens when the stomach's substance, including stomach acid, back up into the throat or mouth. Frequently, this outcome in an acrid or severe taste. In serious cases, spewing forth will cause retching.

Although spewing forth is the most widely recognized side effect, a few different symptoms could be because of acid reflux. These incorporate

- ✓ Asthma
- ✓ Chest torment
- ✓ Cough
- ✓ Dental disintegration
- ✓ Difficulty gulping
- ✓ Excess spit
- ✓ Hoarseness
- ✓ Sore throat

HEARTBURN, ACID REFLUX, AND GERD DURING PREGNANCY

Indigestion, likewise called heartburn or acid reflux, is normal in pregnancy. It tends to be brought about by hormonal changes and the developing child squeezing against your stomach.

You can help facilitate your indigestion and heartburn by making changes to your diet and way of life, and some medicines are sheltered to take in pregnancy.

The reverse of stomach acid into the throat that causes disturbance and consuming sensation in the chest is alluded to as acid reflux or gastroesophageal reflux disease (GERD). There are a few reasons that can cause acid reflux, and the expansion in acid reverse is identified with a blend of our diet, way of life, and heftiness. This condition can influence the two men just as ladies, and the symptoms of acid reflux are commonly the same in people. Pregnant ladies are progressively powerless to acid reflux, particularly in the second and third trimesters.

Acid reflux is a significant basic condition in pregnant ladies. Almost 20 percent of ladies experience heart consume and indigestion in the initial three months of pregnancy. The number hops to 45 percent in the subsequent trimester and around 70 percent in the last three months. Expanded hormonal level, being one of the most widely recognized causes. This is primarily in light of the fact that the expanded degrees of the hormone progesterone, during pregnancy, influence the working of the muscle, responsible for shutting the throat. A debilitating in this muscle permits the reverse of stomach acids into the throat, causing heartburn and acid reflux. Another reason for acid reflux during pregnancy is the expanded weight in the stomach because of the creating of the undeveloped organism.

The creating hatchling causes weight on the upper digestive tract, constraining the stomach substance into the throat.

It's called heartburn, despite the fact that that consuming inclination in your chest has nothing to do with the heart. Awkward and baffling, it pesters numerous ladies, especially during pregnancy.

The principal question you may have is how to make it stop. You may likewise think about whether medications are ok for your infant. Realize what causes heartburn during pregnancy and what can be done.

Symptoms of indigestion and heartburn

The acid reflux symptoms in ladies who are pregnant are commonly equivalent to in some other individual experiencing this condition. The reverse of stomach acids can harm the coating of the throat and can cause aggravation and inconvenience. Here arethe basic symptoms of acid reflux in pregnant ladies:

Symptoms of indigestion and heartburn include:

- ❖ a consuming sensation or torment in the chest
- ❖ feeling full, overwhelming or enlarged
- ❖ burping or burping
- ❖ feeling or being debilitated
- ❖ bringing up nourishment
- ❖ Nausea
- ❖ Vomiting
- ❖ Indigestion
- ❖ Heartburn
- ❖ Cough
- ❖ Sore throat
- ❖ Difficulty in gulping
- ❖ Regurgitation

Thus, these were a portion of the acid reflux symptoms in pregnant ladies. Ladies, for the most part, experience sickness and regurgitating in the initial three months of pregnancy pursued by heartburn and indigestion in the second and third trimesters. For the most part, the acid reflux symptoms experienced by pregnant ladies are mellow, notwithstanding, they can be extreme at times, causing a ton of agony and distress. Along these lines, here are a few tips for getting pregnant ladies far from acid reflux.

Symptoms, for the most part, please not long after in the wake of eating or drinking, yet there can once in a while be a deferral among eating and creating indigestion.

Things you can do to help with indigestion and heartburn

Changes to your diet and way of life might be sufficient to control your symptoms, especially if they are gentle.

Eat strongly

You're bound to get indigestion in case you're full.

In case you're pregnant, it might be enticing to eat more than you would typically. However, this may not be beneficial for you or your child.

Change your eating and drinking propensities.

You might have the option to control your indigestion with changes to your dietary patterns.

It can eat little meals frequently, as opposed to bigger meals three times each day, and to not eat inside three hours of heading to sleep around evening time.

Eliminating drinks containing caffeine, and foods that are rich, spicy or fatty, can likewise ease symptoms.

Keep upstanding

Sit upright when you eat. This will ease the heat off your stomach.

Quit smoking

Smoking when pregnant can cause indigestion, and can truly influence the strength of you and your unborn infant.

At the point when you smoke, the synthetic substances you breathe in can add to your indigestion. These synthetics can cause the ring of muscle at the lower end of your neck to unwind, which permits stomach acid to return up more effectively. This is known as acid reflux.

Smoking likewise expands the risk of:

❖ your infant being conceived rashly (before week 37 of your pregnancy)
❖ your infant being brought into the world with a low birth weight
❖ sudden newborn child demise disorder (SIDS), or "bed passing."

Avoid liquor

Drinking liquor can cause indigestion. During pregnancy, it can likewise prompt long haul mischief to the child. The Chief Medical Officers of the UK state it's most secure to not drink liquor at all in pregnancy.

When to get restorative assistance

See your birthing assistant or GP on the off chance that you need assistance dealing with your symptoms or if changes to your diet and way of life don't work. They may prescribe prescription to facilitate your symptoms.

You ought to likewise observe your birthing specialist or GP in the event that you have any of the accompanying:

- ❖ Difficulty eating or holding nourishment down
- ❖ Weight misfortune
- ❖ Stomach torments

Your maternity specialist or GP may get some information about your symptoms and look at you by squeezing tenderly on various regions of your chest and stomach to see whether this is difficult.

In case you're taking physician recommended meds.

Address your GP in case you're taking a prescription for another condition, for example, antidepressants, and you figure it might be adding to your indigestion. Your GP might have the option to endorse an elective drug.

Take constantly an endorsed prescription except if you're encouraged to do as such by your GP or another certified human service proficient who's liable for your consideration.

Meds for indigestion and heartburn

Meds for indigestion and heartburn during pregnancy include:

❖ Antacids – to kill the acid in your stomach (some are accessible over the counter from a drug specialist)

- ❖ Alginates – to mitigate indigestion brought about by acid reflux by halting the acid in your stomach returning up your neck

You may possibly need to take antacids and alginates when you start getting symptoms. In any case, your GP may prescribe taking them before symptoms, please – for instance, before a meal or before bed.

In case you're accepting iron enhancements just as antacids, don't take them at the same time. Antacids can prevent iron from being consumed by your body.

In the event that antacids and alginates don't improve your symptoms, your GP may endorse a drug to diminish the measure of acid in your stomach. Two that are generally utilized in pregnancy and not known to be hurtful to an unborn infant are:

- ❖ Ranitidine – a tablet you take two times every day
- ❖ Omeprazole – a tablet you take once per day

Causes of indigestion in pregnancy

Symptoms of indigestion come when the acid in your stomach disturbs your stomach lining or your neck. This causes torment and consuming inclination.

At the point when you're pregnant, you're bound to have indigestion due to:

❖ Hormonal changes
❖ The developing infant pushing on your stomach
❖ The muscles between your stomach and neck unwinding, permitting stomach acid to return up

You might be bound to get indigestion in pregnancy if:

❖ You had indigestion before you were pregnant
❖ You've been pregnant previously
❖ You're in the later phases of pregnancy

Does pregnancy cause heartburn?

Pregnancy expands your risk of heartburn or acid reflux. During the primary trimester, muscles in your throat push nourishment all the more gradually into the stomach, and your stomach takes more time to discharge. This gives your body more opportunity to ingest supplements for the baby. However, it can likewise bring about heartburn.

During the third trimester, the development of your infant can drive your stomach out of its typical position, which can prompt heartburn.

Be that as it may, every lady is extraordinary. Being pregnant doesn't really mean you'll have heartburn. It relies upon numerous variables, including your physiology, diet, every day propensities, and your pregnancy.

Would I be able to make the way of life changes that help make it stop?

Mitigating heartburn during pregnancy normally includes some experimentation. Way of life propensities that can decrease heartburn is frequently the most secure techniques for mother and infant. The accompanying tips may help alleviate your heartburn:

- ❖ Eat little meals all the more as often as possible and avoid drinking while at the same time eating. Savor water between meals.
- ❖ Eat gradually and bite each chomp altogether.
- ❖ Avoid foods and refreshments that trigger your heartburn. Commonplace guilty parties incorporate chocolate, fatty foods, spicy foods, acidic foods like citrus fruits and tomato-based things, carbonated drinks, and caffeine.
- ❖ Stay upstanding for at any rate one hour after a meal. A lackadaisical walk may likewise energize digestion.
- ❖ Wear agreeable as opposed to a tight-fitting dress.
- ❖ Maintain a solid weight.
- ❖ Use cushions or wedges to lift your chest area while dozing.

- ❖ Sleep on your left side. Lying on your correct side will situate your stomach higher than your throat, which may prompt heartburn.
- ❖ Chew a bit of sugarless gum after meals. The expanded salivation may kill any acid returning up into the throat.
- ❖ D yogurt or drink a glass of milk to subdue symptoms once they start.
- ❖ Drink some nectar in chamomile tea or a glass of warm milk.

Elective drug alternatives incorporate needle therapy and unwinding strategies, for example, dynamic muscle unwinding, yoga, or guided symbolism. Continuously check with your PCP before attempting new medicines.

What meds are sheltered to take during pregnancy?

Over-the-counter antacids, for example, Tums, Rolaids, and Maalox, may assist you with adapting to incidental heartburn symptoms. It might be ideal to avoid magnesium during the last trimester of pregnancy. Magnesium could meddle with constrictions during work.

Most specialists suggest avoiding antacids that contain elevated levels of sodium. These antacids can prompt the development of liquid in the tissues. You ought to likewise avoid any antacids that rundown aluminum on the mark, as in "aluminum hydroxide" or "aluminum carbonate." These antacids can prompt stoppage.

At last, avoid meds like Alka-Seltzer that may contain headache medicine.

Approach your PCP for the best alternative. I you end up bringing down jugs of antacids, your heartburn may have advanced to gastroesophageal acid reflux disease (GERD). All things considered, you may require a more grounded treatment.

When would it be a good idea for me to converse with my PCP?

If you have heartburn that frequently awakens you around evening time, returns when your antacid wears off or makes different symptoms (for example, trouble gulping, hacking, weight reduction, or dark stools), you may have an increasingly significant issue that requires consideration. Your primary care physician may determine you to have GERD. This implies your heartburn should be controlled to shield you from complexities, for example, harm to the throat.

Your PCP may recommend certain acid-lessening drugs to diminish your symptoms. Meds called H2 blockers, which help obstruct the creation of acid, have all the earmarks of being protected. Another sort of drug, called proton siphon inhibitors, is utilized for individuals with heartburn that doesn't react to different medicines.

In case you're worried about the impacts of drugs, make certain to converse with your PCP. Specialists can assist you in controlling your symptoms while guarding your unborn child.

ACID REFLUX (GERD) IN CHILDREN: CAUSES, SYMPTOMS, AND TREATMENT

Acid reflux or gastro esophageal reflux (GER) is the automatic entry of gastric substance into the throat. It is typical for a child to have incidental scenes of acid reflux as they, for the most part, stop with a couple of dietary changes. In the event that they happen alongside different confusions, at that point, it is a great idea to counsel a specialist.

Acid Reflux Symptoms In Children

Symptoms of acid reflux in children will shift contingent upon their age. Babies with reflux ordinarily let out nourishment regularly and give indications of diminished craving, rest unsettling influence, and crabbiness. Be that as it may, GERD or genuine acid reflux is exceptionally far-fetched in a generally sound and flourishing baby.

The most normally observed side effect of acid reflux in children more than 12 years old just as more seasoned youngsters is heartburn – a consuming sensation felt behind the breastbone and/or center of mid-region. Much of the time, children who are under 12 years old don't regularly whine of heartburn. In more established children and teenagers, some other acid reflux symptoms include:

- ❖ Discomfort while gulping
- ❖ Frequent hack or wheeze
- ❖ Hoarseness
- ❖ Excessive burping
- ❖ Frequent queasiness
- ❖ Taste of stomach acid in the throat
- ❖ Pain when resting in the wake of eating
- ❖ The feeling of nourishment stuck in the throat.

In little youngsters and preschoolers, symptoms of acid reflux can be:

- ❖ Poor craving (a few guardians notice their child lean towards fluids to strong nourishment)
- ❖ Regurgitation
- ❖ Weight Loss
- ❖ Nausea
- ❖ Vomiting
- ❖ Bad Breath
- ❖ Pain during Swallowing
- ❖ Tooth Erosion brought about by acid support up into the mouth.
- ❖ Chronic Cough or Sore Throat
- ❖ Respiratory Problems like Wheezing or intermittent Pneumonia

The great symptoms of acid reflux in children include:

- ❖ Nausea and successive disgorging and regurgitating very quickly in the wake of eating something

- ❖ Regular heartburn, for example, a consuming and difficult sensation in the chest, behind the breastbone, and a consuming sensation in the stomach (in children 12 years and up)
- ❖ Pain when you swallow, trouble gulping
- ❖ Refusal to eat
- ❖ Bad breath
- ❖ An acrid preference for the mouth, particularly in the mornings
- ❖ Choking and gasping, when nourishment enters the windpipe.

The point at which Acid Reflux Becomes Gastroesophageal Reflux Disease (GERD)

If your child is encountering acid reflux for more than two times every week constantly for half a month, at that point, it could be GERD. It is an increasingly extreme condition and might require a specialist's determination.

Appropriate Time To Take Your Child To The Doctor.

As per the University of Rochester Medical Center, call the specialist promptly if your child:

- ❖ Vomits a great deal and/or it contains blood
- ❖ Has breathing issue, wheezing and hacking
- ❖ Shows indications of lack of hydration
- ❖ Has shed pounds

A portion of the essential symptoms of acid reflux may likewise demonstrate other minor infirmities. So you may not surge your child to the specialist on the off chance that the individual in question heaves a bit, grumbles of a stomach throb, or will not eat on occasion. However, on the off chance that these symptoms are reliable and visit, it is a reason for concern and warrants an outing to the specialist.

Causes Of Acid Reflux In Children

Acid reflux in children may happen when the lower esophageal sphincter (LES) unwinds over and over again or takes too long to even think about relaxing. It causes stomach acid to stream back to the throat.

If your child has infrequent acid reflux, at that point, it may be because of some way of life issues, for example,

- ❖ Obesity
- ❖ Overeating
- ❖ Having a greater amount of citrus, chocolate, fatty and spicy foods
- ❖ Consuming liquor (on account of adolescents)
- ❖ Long-term use of headache medicine and a couple of over-the-counter nonsteroidal calming medications, for example, ibuprofen and naproxen.
- ❖ Allergic state of the throat

Intermittent acid reflux could stop with some way of life changes. In any case, if acid reflux is extreme and happens all the more much of the time, at that point, the reason could lie further.

Causes Of GERD In Children

A couple of causes for GERD may be:

- ❖ Neurological impedance, for example, cerebral paralysis, which influences body developments and muscle coordination.
- ❖ The neuromuscular issue, for example, innate myopathy, which is a birth imperfection that causes dynamic muscle shortcoming.
- ❖ Trachea-esophageal fistula medical procedure, which is a restorative medical procedure for birth absconds in the throat and trachea.
- ❖ Genetic conditions, for example, Trisomy 21, which is a state of having an extra chromosome. Another condition is having a solid family ancestry of GERD.
- ❖ Congenital diaphragmatic hernia, which is birth deserts in the stomach muscles.

❖ Lung diseases, for example, asthma and bronchiectasis.

❖ Significant rashness, which happens when infants are conceived before 28 weeks of pregnancy.

Your primary care physician is the best individual to evaluate and analyze your child. In the following segment, we enlighten you concerning a portion of the techniques specialists may use to analyze acid reflux or GERD.

Diagnosing Acid Reflux Or GERD In Children

The specialist would initially check for the symptoms referenced previously. The medicinal history of the child and development diagram is frequently enough for the specialist to analyze GERD in children. Now and again, further tests might be prescribed. They include:

❖ A pH test, which is an entangled test that decides the acid levels in the throat.

❖ Gastric purging examination

❖ Upper GI endoscopy, to glimpse inside the stomach, throat and the small digestive system

How to Diagnose GERD in A Child?

If your child is of the age where he can discuss his concern with the specialist, at that point, the specialist will pose different inquiries to your child, do a physical assessment and get some information about different symptoms as well. This data will enable the specialist to choose the right course of treatment for your child. If your infant or more youthful child is the casualty of this issue, at that point your PCP may direct after assessment to affirm the finding:

1. Milk Scans: Milk check or gastric purging investigation that includes receiving x-beam methods to screen the fluid in the child's stomach. This test builds up if the fluid is getting breathed into the lungs or stomach is acting gradually in purging the fluid.

2. Upper GI Test Or Barium Test: This is a test that shows how the throat responds to barium. It helps in recognizing any variations from the norm or bothering in the throat.

3. pH Probe Or 24-hour Impedance-Probe Study: This is an obtrusive system where a slight adaptable cylinder embedded through the nose into the throat to check the acid levels.

4. Upper GI Endoscopy: In this system, a minor camera is utilized to see legitimately into the throat, stomach, and the small digestive tract to see for the reasonable justification of acid reflux.

Potential Complications of Pediatric GERD

GERD or gastroesophageal reflux disease may, in some cases, cause genuine intricacy in children. Following are a portion of the entanglements that may emerge:

- ❖ It may mess breathing up in children. This may happen when the stomach's substance enters the trachea, nose, or lungs of the child.
- ❖ Sometimes GERD may cause seeping in the throat.
- ❖ Some children may create esophagitis, a condition coming about because of aggravation and redness of the throat.
- ❖ In a few cases, children may create scar tissue in the throat. This may make gulping very hard for the child.

Treatment For Children Suffering from Acid Reflux And GERD

Beginning from an essential way of life and diet changes to prescriptions, treatment for acid reflux and GERD relies upon the seriousness of the symptoms. For more youthful children, specialists, as a rule, prescribe changes in diet and way of life to avert setting off the turmoil. Here are some of them:

- ❖ Eat all the more regularly, however, eat littler meals each time. Avoid eating, at any rate, three hours before sleep time.
- ❖ If the child is large, weight reduction is prescribed to diminish any conceivable weight on the midriff.
- ❖ Keep the head in a raised position when resting, and likes to rest towards the left side.
- ❖ Avoid wearing tight garments.
- ❖ Do not eat enormous or substantial meals before enthusiastic exercise, a game, or some other upsetting occasion.

Notwithstanding these tips, the specialist may likewise endorse acid reflux drug, for example,

- ❖ Antacids
- ❖ Proton siphon inhibitors like Nexium, Prevacid
- ❖ Histamine-2 blockers to help decrease the acid in the stomach

Careful treatment may be prescribed to children with interminable backsliding GERD, and when all the elective treatment alternatives neglect to give help (5).

Recollect that these drugs ought not to be taken without the specialist's recommendation.

Foods to Prevent Gastroesophageal Reflux Disease in Child

There are numerous triggers of acid reflux, and thinking about them will assist you with keeping your child's concern under control. Here are some nourishment things that you ought not to let your child need to forestall gastroesophageal reflux:

- ❖ Oily, spicy, and fatty nourishment things.
- ❖ Chocolates and sugary foods.
- ❖ Mint or peppermint
- ❖ Any citrus fruits, for example, organs, lemons, sweet limes, and so forth.
- ❖ Tomatoes and any dish arranged with tomatoes.
- ❖ Caffeinated drinks

❖ Onions and garlic

Characteristic Remedies For Acid Reflux In Children

In any case, these may not fix reflux and can't supplant a specialist's recommendation. Accept your primary care physician's recommendation before attempting any of these remedies for your children.

1. Yogurt

Eating yogurt may support reflux. Studies have demonstrated that the aging of milk produces bioactive peptides, which could help in securing the gut divider.

Instructions to: Give the child a large portion of a cup of plain crisp yogurt consistently after a meal.

2. Sugarless gum

Biting gum may help increment the gulping recurrence, accordingly improving the leeway pace of throat.

Step by step instructions to Giving your child sugarless biting gum after a meal may help in lessening acid reflux.

3. Fennel seeds

Other than being a superb digestive, fennel seeds may likewise help in decreasing acidity. The seeds have a protein called anethole, which has antispasmodic properties that may help in lessening acid reflux.

Step by step instructions to If your child is mature enough to bite, at that point, give them a spoonful of fennel seeds to bite after meals.

4. Aniseed and cumin seed

It is said that aniseed soothingly affects a disturbed stomach, so it may be useful to lessen acid reflux.

Step by step instructions to:

❖ Get the child to bite some aniseed in the wake of eating nourishment.

❖ Alternatively, drench the aniseed alongside sugar candy in some water for three to four hours. Strain the water and offer it to the child to drink.

❖ You can likewise consider utilizing aniseed glue to egg and meat dishes to help digest it appropriately, and counteract any heartburn.

Moreover, cumin seeds can be utilized to treat acid reflux in children. Other than utilizing them in your nourishment (Indian dishes), you can likewise get the child to bite these seeds on the off chance that he has a consuming sensation in the stomach.

5. Ginger root

Ginger root could be utilized for diminishing acid reflux. Concentrates found that ginger root improved gastric purging and gastroduodenal versatility in fasting and nourished state (9).

The most effective method to:

- ❖ Clean a bit of ginger, strip, and mesh it. Concentrate the juice from it and blend it in with a glass of warm water. Offer it to the child to drink on a vacant stomach.
- ❖ You can likewise utilize ginger in nourishment to anticipate acid reflux symptoms.

6. Aloe vera

Concentrates found that aloe vera is a protected and powerful treatment for decreasing the symptoms of GERD.

Step by step instructions to:

- ❖ Slit an aloe vera cylinder and take the gel out from it. Add that gel to water and bubble it.

7. Basil leaves

Basil or Tulsi leaves are accepted to be powerful in treating the symptoms of acid

8. Apple juice vinegar

There is no logical proof to demonstrate its viability; episodic proof recommends that it may work to lessen acid reflux.

The most effective method to: Combine one teaspoon of ACV with a large portion of a glass of water and offer it to him in the first part of the day. This will help reestablish the pH balance in the stomach.

9. Coconut oil

Coconut oil has mitigating properties and might help decrease the irritation caused because of acid reflux. In any case, inquire about says that coconut oil ought to be devoured in.

The most effective method to Give one teaspoon of coconut oil to the child once per day. YBe that as it may, ensure your child isn't hypersensitive and likewise counsel with your primary care physician before managing coconut oil orally to your child.

These home remedies help in easing the symptoms of acid reflux, yet not restoring it altogether.

Foods To Avoid To Prevent Acid Reflux

Is milk useful for acid reflux? Will my children eat candy when they have acid reflux? What would they be able to eat to anticipate acid reflux?

❖ chocolate

❖ Mint

❖ Spicy, slick, or oily foods – avoid a wide range of quick foods.

❖ Tomatoes or anything produced using tomatoes.

❖ Citrus fruits, for example, oranges, lemon, and so on.

Attempt and give the child just custom made foods beyond what many would consider possible. Control or point of confinement the segments, as gorging can likewise trigger sickness and retching related to acid reflux. If the specialist has recommended any prescriptions, check on the off chance that it is alright to utilize these home remedies alongside the drugs.

Reflux Medication Is Not Always The Answer

With regards to utilizing reflux drugs in children to stifle gastric acid creation, the extraordinary alert must be utilized. Studies find that PPIs or Proton Pump Inhibitors (which are fairly usually endorsed by most pediatricians) are not powerful in lessening GERD symptoms in newborn children. Fake treatment controlled preliminaries in more seasoned children are inadequate. Although PPIs appear to be all around endured during momentary use, proof supporting the security of PPIs is deficient. Additionally, PPIs can burglarize the assortment of basic supplements; these medications don't treat the condition at its root and just give alleviation from prompt symptoms.

A few specialists can recommend PPIs for children who have both asthma and GERD with the expectation that smothering gastric acid will show upgrades in symptoms of the two diseases, yet this couldn't be further away from reality. An investigation done in Norway found that treatment with normal PPIs to smother acid generation didn't improve asthma symptoms or lung work in children with asthma and GERD.

Long haul utilization of acid meds can cause genuine symptoms, as:

- ❖ Lead to press, zinc, calcium, nutrient B12 and magnesium insufficiency
- ❖ Increased risk of intense gastroenteritis and network gained pneumonia in children.
- ❖ Increase the risk of constant kidney disease
- ❖ Increase the odds of parasitic infections in the gut
- ❖ Increase risk of enteric infections
- ❖ Increase the risk of cracks
- ❖ Alter the bacterial greenery of the upper gastrointestinal tract

- ❖ Reduce sound gut microscopic organisms while expanding terrible, disease-causing microorganisms in the gut
- ❖ Lead to Clostridia difficile infections, which is a difficult-to-treat microscopic organism causing diarrhea
- ❖ Cause bacterial infections of the small digestion tracts

Breakfast Foods to Eat with Acid Reflux

Breakfast has consistently been hailed as the most significant meal of the day. It turns out this familiar maxim is out and out obvious, particularly for acid reflux sufferers. Topping off the stomach with great nourishment can counteract acid assaults for the duration of the day and mitigate symptoms of acid reflux.

What sort of breakfast foods are appropriate for individuals with acid reflux? The thought is to eat antacid foods that won't add to or trigger reflux symptoms. This incorporates oatmeals, select fruits, and vegetables, just as lean protein.

If you experience the ill effects of serious or incessant acid reflux, otherwise called gastroesophageal reflux disease (GERD), you might be animated to alter your diet. The customary American breakfast incorporates a few things that could trigger symptoms. Be that as it may, everybody's resilience of foods is unique. Instead of consequently precluding specific things, the American College of Gastroenterology's 2013 clinical practice rules prescribes an individual methodology - that you decide for yourself what foods exasperate your symptoms. Certain decisions, be that as it may, are bound to trigger acid reflux, and on the off chance that you find conventional breakfast things are raising you ruckus, despite everything you have numerous energizing other options.

Espresso, Tea, and Milk

In the event that you like espresso or tea toward the beginning of the day, you might be sufficiently blessed to endure these without acid reflux symptoms. Notwithstanding, these refreshments may possibly intensify symptoms by loosening up the band of muscles called the lower esophageal sphincter, or LES, that fills in as an obstruction valve between the throat and the stomach. At the point when the LES unwinds, acidic digestive juices spill into the throat, causing aggravation and disturbance. Other potential triggers to acid reflux symptoms incorporate mint tea, hot cocoa, other charged refreshments, and drinks containing liquor. Natural teas might be a non-bothering elective. For instance, chamomile's calming advantages may support the agony and aggravation of GERD. Milk is normally all-around endured, albeit low-fat or nonfat milk might be preferable alternatives over entire milk. Soluble foods - including plant-based kinds of milk, for example, almond and soy - may likewise diminish stomach acidity, albeit more research is expected to decide the viability of this methodology.

Fruits and Juices

Fruits and squeezes are regular breakfast decisions and, whenever endured, sound increments to the morning meal. Be that as it may, certain fruits and squeezes are viewed as acidic -, for example, citrus fruits, and tomato juice - and devouring these might trigger acid reflux symptoms by disturbing a previously excited throat. The acid in these foods can likewise initiate pepsin, the compound found in gastric liquids, which is answerable for protein breakdown. Any pepsin initiated in the throat could harm its covering. Consequently, it's a smart thought to avoid fruits or squeezes that irritate your symptoms. Apples, bananas, avocados, watermelon, melon, and pears are instances of lower acid fruits that may work better.

Pieces of Bread and Cereals

Bread and oats are staples in most breakfast meals. When in doubt, these foods are very much endured and don't bother acid reflux symptoms. Be that as it may, high-fat decisions, for example, croissants, doughnuts, sweet rolls, and biscuits, may slow stomach discharging - and the substance of a full stomach is bound to reflux into the throat. High fiber breakfast decisions, for example, entire grain bread, entire wheat English biscuits, wheat oat, or oatmeal, are better choices - they are normally low in fat, and the fiber helps move nourishment all the more rapidly however the digestive framework. In the event that you increment your fiber consumption rapidly, you can incidentally endure more gas and swelling, so it's ideal to step by step fuse more fiber into your diet.

Breakfast Proteins

Protein foods, for example, eggs, curds, nutty spread, and breakfast meats, are regular breakfast decisions.

High-fat meat items, for example, bacon or frankfurter, may hinder stomach discharging, and this can compound acid reflux by loosening up the LES and expanding acid generation in the stomach. Eggs are commonly all around endured, yet are best arranged bubbled, poached or cooked in a nonstick dish with almost no oil. More slender meat choices incorporate Canadian bacon, ham, and turkey or chicken frankfurter. Likewise, consider plant-based choices, for example, nut or almond margarine, delicately mixed tofu, soy bacon strips, and soy frankfurter joins.

Contemplations and Precautions

Acid reflux and GERD are overseen by a blend of drug treatment and lifestyle changes. While no foods are generally confined for acid reflux sufferers, certain diet techniques may help ease symptoms. Losing overabundance weight is a successful method to control, and even counteract acid reflux symptoms, so a less fatty, more beneficial breakfast is a decent spot to begin. On the off chance that any foods or refreshments exacerbate your acid reflux, think about constraining or avoiding them. You can likewise limit your symptoms by not resting a few hours in the wake of eating. At long last, make certain to have breakfast, on the grounds that skipping meals may provoke you to gorge later - and a full stomach can irritate symptoms. If not oversaw well, acid reflux and GERD can prompt genuine complexities, including the risk of esophageal malignancy. Tell your primary care physician if acid reflux is genuinely affecting your personal satisfaction, particularly if you are encountering chest torment, interminable hack, or wheezing.

Signs You Have Acid Reflux

Burping? Blockage? Stomach cramps? You may believe you're simply encountering morning cravings for food when you're really encountering acid reflux.

Acid reflux is a typical issue that happens when a muscle called the lower esophageal sphincter (LES) neglects to seal in stomach juices. At the point when the LES unwinds or glitches, stomach acid can move back up the throat, causing consuming in the throat joined by an acrid taste.

Different indications of acid reflux include:

- ❖ Nausea
- ❖ Burping and hiccups
- ❖ Bloating
- ❖ Regurgitation; tasting harsh or acrid tasting acid with each burp
- ❖ Bad breath
- ❖ Chest torment
- ❖ Burning sensation on the chest

In what capacity Can Food Trigger Acid Reflux?

There is no reasonable evidence that specific nutritional categories can cause acid reflux; it is realized that particular foods can trigger or disturb existing symptoms.

Nourishment can be utilized to limit the acidity of stomach substance by modifying the diet as needs are. A few foods can even reason the LES to unwind, which could compound the spewing forth of stomach acids.

6 Breakfast No-Nos: What to Avoid

1. Foods with high-fat substance

Studies show that individuals who expend nourishment with elevated levels of cholesterol and immersed fat are likelier to encounter acid reflux symptoms (source). Fatty foods take more time to separate than their more beneficial partners. The stomach is compelled to deliver progressively acid so as to appropriately process these foods, prompting heartburn.

Foods considered high in fat incorporate anything southern style. Ham, bacon, french fries, onion rings, and pretty much anything trickling with oil are clear instances of foods to avoid while encountering acid reflux.

2. Caffeine

Caffeine, both in espresso and caffeinated drinks, ought to be avoided by acid reflux sufferers. Caffeine is known to loosen up the LES, causing acid reflux. However, this fluctuates, relying upon an individual's digestive tract. High measures of caffeine likewise mean higher acidity, which can additionally disturb a previously bothered digestive framework.

Notwithstanding, it's as yet conceivable to appreciate some espresso toward the beginning of the day without prompting heartburn. First off, you could investigate espresso choices that have a lower caffeine substance, for example, decaffeinated espresso and a latte.

Choosing low-caffeine drink options; for example, tea is likewise a feasible breakfast choice. Note that a few teas are really acidic in nature. Mint-based may intensify reflux symptoms.

3. Spicy foods

Spicy foods are remembered for the National Institute of Diabetes and Digestive and Kidney Diseases rundown of foods that decline acid reflux. Spicy foods are referred to go about as aggravations that may diminish LES usefulness, prompting heartburn. These likewise support the creation of stomach acid, which doesn't support an effectively uninvolved LES.

4. Chocolate

Chocolate contains certain segments that aggravate the stomach, for example, caffeine, theobromine, and methylxanthine. It is essential fixing, cocoa powder, is likewise acidic in nature. Then again, a few chocolates might be all the more obliging to a delicate stomach.

5. Acidic fruits, vegetables, and fixings

While fruits and vegetables are by and large prescribed to any diet, acid reflux sufferers ought to be careful about expending a lot of specific foods. These incorporate oranges, grapefruits, lemons, limes, tomatoes, pineapple, and whatever other nourishment that is high in acidity.

Results of these fruits and vegetables, including lemoned, unadulterated organic product juices, and salsa, ought to be expended with some restraint or avoided through and through.

6. Skirting the Most Important Meal of the Day

The demonstration of having breakfast alone is known to help oversee interminable acid reflux. By eating something toward the beginning of the day, acid reflux sufferers give their void stomachs something to process. Rather than going up the throat, the acids can take a shot at solid breakfast nourishment, decreasing sentiments of clogging and stomach cramps.

Eating promptly toward the beginning of the day can likewise quiet the stomach and forestall symptoms for the duration of the day. Then again, skipping breakfast is known to both prompt and intensify acid reflux symptoms.

Top Breakfast Foods For Fighting Acid Reflux

Planning meals may feel all the more testing when eating with acid reflux sufferers. Be that as it may, there are as yet nourishment choices accessible for individuals with even the most touchy of stomachs:

Soluble Fruits and Vegetables.

Apples, bananas, coconuts, apricots, avocados, pears, and blueberries are instances of soluble fruits. Swap out acidic fruits for these and include them as toppers for your oat, oatmeal, or flapjack.

Potato, squash, and zucchini are among the morning meal cordial, antacid vegetables. Squash and prepare these vegetables together to make sound potato tots.

Oatmeal

Oatmeal is a stunning power food with practically zero acidic substance. Oatmeal keeps you more full for more, is anything but difficult to process, and is fantastically nutritious. Blend in some almond milk or a large portion of some skim milk for included flavor. Include low-acid fruits, for example, apples and bananas, to make your oatmeal somewhat more uncommon.

Ginger

Ginger gloats of mitigating properties that can improve nourishment digestion and counteract post-meal acid reflux. Swap out your morning espresso and tea for soaks ginger tea. Finish off with a spoon of nectar.

Verdant Greens

Vegetables, for example, spinach, lettuce, and kale, can be changed into a solid breakfast meal. Prepare a bubbled egg and some chicken bits with some destroyed lettuce to make a tasty breakfast serving of mixed greens. Spinach and kale can be hacked, alongside mushrooms and peas, for a yummy morning omelet. Verdant greens are low-acid, high-volume foods that will help kill acid in the stomach.

Chicken and turkey

Lean protein, for example, chicken and turkey, make extraordinary breakfast meals. To protect lean meat for acid reflux sufferers, consider heating them in a stove as opposed to hurling them in a skillet.

Almond or Soy Milk

Grain, oatmeal, and breakfast biscuits don't need to be exhausting. Including a sprinkle of almond milk or soy milk can take breakfast to an unheard-of level. Observe that not all nut-based milk has a similar pH.

Cashew milk, for example, is viewed as acid-framing nourishment and may actuate acid reflux at breakfast.

Breakfast Recipes for Acid Reflux

Dairy-Free Pancake

Fixings:

- ❖ 1 cup of universally handy flour
- ❖ 2 teaspoons heating powder
- ❖ 1 cup unsweetened almond milk
- ❖ 1 huge egg
- ❖ 1 huge egg yolk
- ❖ 1 ½ teaspoon canola oil
- ❖ 2 tablespoons sugar
- ❖ 1 can splash cooking oil

Instructions:

1. Add wet ingredients and dry ingredients on the other hand. Continue blending until all substance are joined

2. Spray skillet with oil at that point pour the blend

3. Cook until delicate darker or no air pockets are appearing

Omelet

Ingredients:

- ❖ 2 enormous eggs
- ❖ Minced mushrooms (or some other antacid vegetable)
- ❖ Diced spinach (or some other verdant green)
- ❖ Salt and pepper to taste

Instructions

1. Whisk the two eggs into a bowl, at that point, include vegetables. You may likewise decide to dark-colored the vegetables for 5 minutes before adding them to the egg blend

2. Heat oil in a container

3. Pour blend and trust that the omelet will shape

No-Bake Faux Banana Bread

Ingredients:

- ❖ 4 huge ready bananas
- ❖ 1 huge egg
- ❖ 2 tbsp. nectar (discretionary)
- ❖ 1 can splash oil
- ❖ 1 tbsp.p.cinnamon powder

Instructions:

1. Mash ready bananas onto a bowl, at that point, include egg. Whisk together. Include cinnamon powder and nectar

2. Spray container with oil

3. Pour blend into the container and sit tight for it to frame

Potato Tots

Ingredients:

- ❖ ¼ cup carrots
- ❖ ¼ cup sweet potato
- ❖ ¼ squash

- ❖ 1 tablespoon flour
- ❖ Salt and pepper to taste

Instructions:

1. Preheat broiler to 450 degrees Fahrenheit

2. Peel and bubble carrots, sweet potato, and squash. At the point when a delicate, channel, and shred

3. Mix vegetables with flour, salt, and pepper

4. Form into little balls and heat for 20 minutes or until brilliant darker

Making Breakfast Easy: Tips For Acid Reflux Sufferers

Tip #1: Keep a Food Diary. Not all foods make similar responses in individuals. Trial with specific foods and see which ones bother your symptoms. Knowing how certain morning meal foods associate with your stomach makes it simpler to design meals later on.

Tip 2: Don't Lie Immediately After Eating. Take a walk or sit up and utilize the PC. Resting can cause indigestion, which can exacerbate acid reflux.

Tip #3: Take Antacids. Over-the-counter antacids are accessible to help keep acid assaults under control. Take a prescribed portion subsequent to having breakfast to avert stomach substance from going up the throat.

Tip #4: Eat Less, More Frequently. Gorging is a trigger of acid reflux. Eating less more as often as possible can keep a touchy digestive framework from delivering an excess of stomach acid at once. Eat little snacks in the middle of meals or separation a major breakfast into two littler servings/

Tip #5: Look For Alternatives. Are there sure breakfast staples you can't manage without? It's as yet conceivable to appreciate them by distinguishing key ingredients that make the nourishment acidic.

Eating the correct sort of breakfast is only one-way patients can monitor acid reflux.

THE MOST EFFECTIVE METHOD TO TREAT BAD BREADTH FROM ACID REFLUX

Acid reflux and terrible breath typically go hand-in-hand. However, the reason for acid reflux, just as some prompt remedies you can apply right presently to improve your breath.

How would you treat awful breath from acid reflux? Restorative mediation is typically applied to further developed cases, yet making a way of life changes are incredible for getting long haul results. Stopping smoking, constraining liquor and caffeine utilization, and taking antacids are, for the most part, extraordinary approaches to mitigate acid reflux and counteract terrible breath.

Acid reflux, as a rule, happens when stomach acids bubble up to the throat, the cylinder moving nourishment starting from the mouth to the stomach.

A muscle called the gastroesophageal sphincter is answerable for keeping stomach acid right where it has a place. In any case, certain triggers can cause the "valve" to glitch, and the acid is brought back up to the throat. Different substances, including bile and undigested nourishment particles, can likewise advance toward the throat.

Albeit normal, acid reflux can form into an interminable condition. Persevering acid reflux symptoms that show more than two times per week will be described as GERD or gastroesophageal reflux disease. Now, doctors may prescribe medicinal intercession to deal with the disease.

Could acid reflux give you awful breath?

Besides heartburn, the most widely recognized grumbling of patients encountering acid reflux is awful breath. Stomach substance may spew back to the throat, including any stomach acids, bile, and undigested nourishment that will wait in your throat and creep up your pharynx, causing awful breath.

Will acid reflux cause you to smell your own terrible breath?

Acids joining to the dividers of your throat can be smelled by others. This is on the grounds that gas particles can likewise join to the tongue, which can irritate the awful stench. Patients with acid reflux frequently report burping, which can likewise increase the smell of stomach acid.

Then again, acid reflux breath may likewise be smelled by the patient. Sometimes, patients report smelling their very own breath even without opening their mouths. Bile drifts from the stomach up to the nose, which delivers a sharp, frequently acidic smell.

What does acid reflux breath smell like?

Acid reflux all alone scents like bile. Anything sulfuric, impactful, solid, and acidic can be described as an acid reflux smell. Patients likewise report various scents dependent on the prescription they are taking to oversee GERD.

Any kind of smell present in the mouth can be symptomatic of ulcers and other gastrointestinal problems. We prescribe getting looked at by a gastroenterologist to administer acid reflux and other potential diseases.

Indications that Acid Reflux Caused Your Bad Breath

Terrible breath is commonly overseen by flossing, brushing the teeth, and utilizing mouthwash. Nonetheless, progressively determined instances of awful breath could point to problems that don't have anything to do with the mouth.

Here are a few signs that awful breath is being brought about by acid reflux:

1. It's identified with nourishment. At the point when awful breath appears to pursue any eating example, it might be a direct result of gastrointestinal problems. Regardless of whether it's eating excessively or excessively small, eating spicy or sharp nourishment, the fact of the matter is that the terrible breath is activated by an encouraging example.

At the point when you see that the terrible breath comes subsequent to drinking espresso, it may be the case that the acid in the espresso is activating stomach acids, prompting awful reflux. Test out your breath subsequent to eating certain foods and check whether any nourishing propensities trigger a terrible breath.

2. It corresponds with other digestive symptoms. Obstruction, swelling, burping, and agony would all be able to be indications of acid reflux. This is

particularly obvious when digestive symptoms come directly after an encouraging example.

In the wake of drinking espresso, do you experience squeezes in your lower stomach area? Do you start burping and experience a solid metallic preference for your mouth? Focusing on your body's physical responses to nourishment is a powerful method for precluding the reason for awful breath.

3. Your breath smells acrid or acidic. Bile is generally portrayed as acridity joined by a copying sensation. Stomach acid reverse into the throat, for the most part, comes as bile, which is a particular indication of acid reflux and indigestion.

4. It deteriorates with caffeine, liquor, and tobacco use. Acid reflux is brought about by the gastroesophageal sphincter debilitating, prompting spewing forth of stomach substance back to the throat.

Ingredients in stimulated and alcoholic items are known to debilitate the gastroesophageal sphincter. Different foods, for example, chocolate, foods high in fat and acid, just as mint, onions, and garlic, may deliver a similar response.

5. You feel inconvenience in your throat. The acid reverse is typically going with a solid acidic sensation in the throat, definitely on the grounds that the acid isn't intended to happen outside the stomach.

In the event that your throat feels scratchy, bothersome, or tingly subsequent to burping, these are clear indications of acid reflux. A consuming sensation in the throat joined by awful stench is a telling sign you have stomach problems.

6. Your tonsils are influenced. A few patients may intuitively visit their dental specialist for a conference subsequent to finding that they have terrible breath. Dental specialists can give a primer conclusion by precluding the reason for terrible breath.

Irritation around the throat, together with acid disintegration on the teeth, are signs to keep an eye out for. Your dental specialist may prescribe a visit to a doctor after the dental test once indications of disturbance are found.

Bad Breath And Acid Reflux

Acid reflux itself isn't the purpose of awful breath. There are two different ways this circumstance could exasperate the malodorous symptoms, and cause longer scenes of foul oral breath:

1. Tooth Decay: The stomach might be presented to these solid acids, yet it is likewise fixed with a defensive obstruction that prevents the acid from "consuming" the stomach. Be that as it may, different pieces of the body don't have this coating and will be defenseless to acid harm, given delayed presentation.

After some time, acid drifting up through the throat and to the mouth can make teeth gradually disintegrate and spoil. The development of rotting matter around the teeth could add to the awful stench, particularly after the teeth decays. Keep up legitimate oral cleanliness to avoid plaque and microscopic organisms aggregation on and between your teeth.

2. Microorganisms In Mouth and Throat: The throat is intended to be a roadway for the nourishment from the mouth to the stomach. With acid reflux, there is a retrogressive stream or particles that are not intended to remain in the throat.

At the point when left untreated, microscopic organisms can develop on the dividers of the throat, prompting terrible breath. Aggravation, irritation, and a shivering sensation are indications of microscopic organisms nearness in the throat.

Home Remedies for Acid Reflux Breath

- ❖ Observe great oral cleanliness
- ❖ Drink pineapple juice
- ❖ Consume a great deal of water

- ❖ Have some solid yogurt to advance great microscopic organisms development
- ❖ Drink milk to check terrible breath
- ❖ Eat a cut of orange or lemon after meals.
- ❖ Use items with zinc to keep the awful breath under control
- ❖ Drink green tea
- ❖ Snack with apples
- ❖ Make a handcrafted mouthwash with vinegar or heating pop.

Treating Bad Breath from Acid Reflux

One conclusive approach to treat terrible breath is to treat the reason for acid reflux. Triggers can be anything from a straightforward way of life decisions to treatable gastrointestinal problems. Normal causes include:

- ❖ Way of life
- ❖ Being fat
- ❖ Lying down following meals
- ❖ Snacking near sleep time
- ❖ Eating foods that are exceptionally acidic.

❖ Consuming a lot of fatty, fried, or spicy foods

Medicinal

❖ Patients with hiatal hernia are known to encounter acid reflux. This happens when the upper piece of the stomach lumps and moves over the stomach.

❖ Pregnant ladies generally experience acid reflux during pregnancy. Symptoms compound through the span of the third trimester, however, they quickly leave after conveyance.

❖ Taking the drug, for example, ibuprofen, muscle relaxers, and circulatory strain controllers.

How To Treating Acid Reflux

Acid reflux, for the most part, leaves alone. Then again, those with incessant acid reflux or GERD might be endorsed with medicine to help with acid reflux. Not all GERD medicine is good with one patient, so it might require a significant stretch of time to locate the correct treatment.

Terrible breath can leave in as meager as seven days as long as three weeks, contingent upon your treatment plan.

Convenient solutions

The ideal approach to dispose of terrible breath brought about by acid reflux is to treat acid reflux itself. Then again, realizing some convenient solutions can assist you with getting through a whole day without stressing over acid reflux breath:

- ❖ Stay hydrated. Continuously have a glass of water by you. Weaken the stomach acid, however much as could be expected by drinking a lot of water.
- ❖ Consider mint and parsley. Both are known to help with the awful breath, so watch out for these trimmings when feasting with individuals.

- Use crude lemon. Lemon help keep the gastroesophageal sphincter close. A cut or two is fine; devouring acid more than would normally be appropriate may exacerbate acid reflux.

- Use antacids to kill stomach acidity. A few antacids are best utilized 20-30 minutes prior to or after a meal. Adhere to clear instructions to make the most out of the prescription.

- Take some deglycyrrhizinated licorice (DGL) bites. DGL bites are known to expand bodily fluid creation, which shields the throat and stomach from the acid introduction. These are likewise commonly endorsed to help with an ulcer, despite the fact that not to the degree that they supplant antacids.

- Don't drink espresso on an unfilled stomach. Make a point to snatch something to eat before expending anything energized or carbonated.

❖ Refrain from indulging. Essentially, eating an excessive amount of can put a great deal of burden on the gastroesophageal sphincter, which can intensify acid reflux. Consume decently and remain from spicy and acidic nourishment until symptoms improve.

ACID REFLUX RECIPES

At the point when you have acid reflux, what and the amount you eat directly affect how you feel. From avoiding your triggers to watching your bit size to helping up your family's top choices, dealing with your diet is a basic piece of dealing with your acid reflux. That is the reason we've accumulated 90+ plans for individuals with GERD and acid reflux simple to make, heavenly, and won't make you feel denied on your GERD diet

Acid reflux formula: Pan burned tilapia

It is regular information that specialists suggest two servings of fish for each week to help keep up great wellbeing, and this GERD neighborly formula is an incredible method to help satisfy that objective. Tilapia is a gentle tasting whitefish that is an incredible wellspring of lean protein, iron, nutrient D, and sound omega 3 fatty acids. For this dish, we sauté the fish in olive oil, which takes only minutes, and then we top it with scrumptious ginger implanted relish of pineapple, red pepper, and cucumbers. Serve it with some long grain rice as an afterthought, and you'll have a snappy and simple meal for a bustling weeknight. It's sound and scrumptious as well!

Makes 4 servings

Ingredients

❖ 1 cup long-grain rice

- ❖ 2 TBSP.P. Pineapple juice
- ❖ 1 TBSP.P.Ground ginger
- ❖ 2 Tbsp. nectar
- ❖ 2 TBSP.P.olives oil
- ❖ 1 pound Pineapple pieces, new or canned
- ❖ 1 little English cucumber, hacked
- ❖ 1/4 cup hacked red sweet pepper*
- ❖ 1 Tbsp. olive oil
- ❖ 4 6-oz tilapia filets

Bearings

1. Cook rice per bundle bearings

2. Mix next four ingredients include salt and pepper

3. Toss with pineapple, cucumber and pepper pieces

4. Heat 1 tbsp. olive oil in an enormous nonstick skillet over medium warmth

5. Season tilapia fillets with salt and pepper, around 1/4 tbsp. each

6. Add to skillet and cook through around 2 to 3 minutes for every side

[166]

7. Serve tilapia beat with relish and rice as an afterthought

Wholesome data per serving:

Calories 485, sat fat 2.3 g, 325 mg Sodium.

* sweet red peppers ought not to trigger acid reflux, particularly with this negligible sum (1/16 cup for each serving).

Acid reflux amicable formula: Asparagus and green bean serving of mixed greens

Asparagus and green beans are stuffed with supplements and are awesome foods that advance great wellbeing and digestion. They are additionally brimming with season hurled with a Dijon mustard vinaigrette in this GERD well-disposed formula. Different ingredients incorporate bacon, eggs, and destroyed carrots, making an exquisite mix for your sense of taste. It's anything but difficult to plan ahead of time, and flavorful on a sweltering summer day. Appreciate!

Formula serves 12

INGREDIENTS

- ❖ 1 pound new asparagus
- ❖ 1 pound French beans, stems expelled
- ❖ 2 TBSP.P.destroyed carrots

- ❖ 3 to 4 cuts turkey bacon, cooked and disintegrated
- ❖ 3 hard-bubbled eggs, cut into quarters
- ❖ 2 TBSP. Dijon mustard
- ❖ 4 TBSP. balsamic vinegar
- ❖ 3 TBSP.P.olive oil
- ❖ Run of salt and pepper

<u>Headings</u>

1. Bring an enormous pot to a bubble and include beans and asparagus, come back to a bubble, at that point lower warmth and stew around 4 minutes until delicate, don't overcook

2. Drain, wash with cold water and chill in the cooler

3. Whisk together the last four ingredients for the vinaigrette, season to taste

4. Chop cooled vegetables, add to a serving of mixed greens bowl, sprinkle with carrots and bacon.

5. Drizzle with vinaigrette and top with eggs

Wholesome data per serving:

(1/twelfth) – Calories 211, Sat Fat 1 g, Sodium 295 mg

Acid Reflux Friendly Recipe: Black Bean Burger

By Rosemary Dowd

Dark beans are pressed with protein and fiber, which makes them a sound expansion to your diet. They are likewise a fantastic low-calorie option in contrast to meat when you are in the state of mind for a "burger." Tortilla chips and cilantro give this formula a southwestern style, which we upgraded with eggs, green pepper, and an assortment of GERD neighborly seasonings. While framing the patties, make certain to pack them together immovably, and chill in the cooler, so they don't self-destruct when flipped. So damp and delectable, even meat-eaters will adore them.

Formula serves 6

INGREDIENTS

- ❖ 2-15 ounce jars dark beans depleted

- ❖ 2 eggs
- ❖ 1/3 cup hacked green pepper
- ❖ 2 TBSP.P. Flour
- ❖ 2 TBSP.P.minced cilantro
- ❖ 1 tbsp. ground cumin
- ❖ 1/2 tbsp. ground coriander
- ❖ 1/4 tbsp. pepper
- ❖ 1/4 tbsp. salt
- ❖ 1/2 cup prepared tortilla chips, squashed
- ❖ 1/4 cup vegetable oil,
- ❖ Separated pineapple cuts
- ❖ A chunk of ice lettuce
- ❖ 6 entire wheat buns

Bearings

1. Line a rimmed preparing sheet with 3 layers of paper towels and spread the depleted beans.

2. In a huge bowl, squash depleted beans, include eggs, flour, seasonings, and squashed tortilla chips.

3. Shape into 6 patties, refrigerate for 60 minutes.

4. Heat 1 tbsp. oil in a nonstick skillet. Cautiously place 3 burgers into the skillet and cook for 5 minutes.

5. Flip and cook for 3 to 4 additional minutes until fresh.

6. Remove and keep warm; rehash with staying 3 burgers.

7. Serve on entire wheat buns with GERD well-disposed toppings, top with pineapple.

Wholesome data per serving:

360 calories, 1 g sat fat, 697 mg sodium.

Banana pecan biscuits

This sweet treat is extraordinary for breakfast in a hurry. Attempt a clump whenever you have bananas that have abided more promising times.

I adjusted this formula from Mark Bittman's How to Cook Everything Banana Bread. It's hands-down the best banana bread I've at any point had. So why upset flawlessness? All things considered, I needed something that was anything but difficult to solidify in singular servings – biscuits – and I required them to be without dairy as a result of some hypersensitivity issues. I swapped coconut oil for the spread in the first formula, which I think supplements the coconut previously utilized in the formula. I additionally utilized all entire wheat flour to build the fiber content. I normally use "White Whole Wheat flour" since it has indistinguishable dietary advantages from other entire wheat flours. However, it has a lot of milder flavor. It works truly well in biscuits, flapjacks, waffles, and so on.

I trust you like biscuits! (And if you need to know the reality, I made two groups a week ago, and not many of them made it into the cooler.)

Makes 18 biscuits

Ingredients

- ❖ 2 c. entire wheat flour
- ❖ 1 t. salt
- ❖ 1/2 t. heating powder
- ❖ 3/4 c. sugar
- ❖ 1/3 c. oil (I utilized coconut oil)
- ❖ 2 eggs
- ❖ 3 ready bananas, squashed with a fork
- ❖ 1 t. vanilla concentrate
- ❖ 1/2 c. cleaved pecans
- ❖ 1/2 c. ground dried unsweetened coconut

Headings

1. Preheat broiler to 375 degrees and oil a biscuit tin or line with cupcake liners.

2. Mix together the dry ingredients.

3. Beat the eggs and blend in with the oil, and pounded bananas.

4. Add the banana blend to the dry ingredients and mix them until joined.

5. Add the vanilla, pecans, and coconut and mix delicately.

6. Spoon the player into the biscuit tins, filling every compartment around 66% full.

7. Bake biscuits for 17-19 minutes until a toothpick embedded into the center of a biscuit confesses all.

8. Remove from the broiler and let biscuits stand for around five minutes in the container before moving them to a cooling rack.

Healthful data (per biscuit):

Calories 218, Fat 9 g, Carbohydrates 23 g, Protein 3 g, Sodium 139 mg

Slow cooker chicken and grain stew

I love cooking with my slow cooker – it's simple and makes the night somewhat less insane. I particularly like making soups and stews in the slow cooker, and this formula is one of my top picks since it's a "put everything in the simmering pot and turn it on" formula. It's additionally entirely versatile, so don't hesitate to change the seasonings to suit your taste, to incorporate herbs you have on hand, or to avoid explicit triggers. It's a colossal hit with everybody in our family, so check out it today around evening time!

Serves 6

Ingredients

- ❖ 2 chicken bosoms
- ❖ 3/4 cup grain
- ❖ 48 oz. low-sodium chicken soup
- ❖ 1 16 oz. sack solidified blended vegetables
- ❖ 1/4 tbsp. garlic powder*
- ❖ 1 little hacked onion*

- ❖ 2 teaspoons Italian flavoring (or a blend of herbs like basil, oregano, and thyme)
- ❖ 2 inlet leaves
- ❖ Pepper to taste
- ❖ Salt to taste
- ❖ 2 cups cleaved child spinach

Headings

1. Put everything aside from the spinach in the simmering pot, ensuring everything is secured with chick stock.

2. Put on the top, set the simmering pot to low, and cook for 5-6 hours until the grain is delicate.

3. Add the spinach throughout the previous 30 minutes of cooking.

4. Remove and dispose of the straight leaves.

5. Remove the chicken bosoms, shred, at that point, join with the soup. (You can simply shred them in the simmering pot on the off chance that they self-destruct of you.)

*If crisp onions or garlic trigger your heartburn symptoms, take a stab at subbing dried out the onion and garlic powder for those things. A few people discover them increasingly mediocre. Or then again overlook the onion and garlic totally – this dish is excusing.

Chicken cutlets with sauteed mushrooms

We eat a ton of boneless, skinless chicken bosoms at our home. They're flexible, simple to get ready, and an extraordinary wellspring of lean protein. We even keep a reserve of cooked chicken bosoms in the cooler for fast and simple meals like servings of mixed greens, pan-sears, and tacos. A couple of months back, I was searching for some new supper thoughts and ran over this formula. It has gotten one of our top choices and is presently part of our ordinary pivot. I, as a rule, serve it with sautéed spinach and a dried-up loaf to sop up the sauce.

This formula incorporates white wine, which can mess up certain individuals with GERD. In case you're one of them, don't hesitate to substitute chicken stock. I've made this with both relying upon what I have on hand, and it's a hit in any case. I trust you like it!

P.S. The scraps make tasty sandwiches. Simply heat the chicken and mushrooms in the microwave, top with a cut of cheddar, and serve on an entire wheat bun.

Serves 4

Ingredients

- ❖ 1 pound boneless, skinless chicken bosoms (or chicken bosom cutlets)
- ❖ 1/3 cup entire wheat flour
- ❖ 2 tablespoons olive oil
- ❖ 3 tablespoons spread
- ❖ 2 cups mushrooms, cut
- ❖ 1/4 cup of white wine
- ❖ Salt and pepper to taste

Bearings

1. Slice the chicken bosoms down the middle across, so you have slight bits of chicken, and cut back any abundance excess. (Avoid this progression in case you're utilizing cutlets.)

2. Season the chicken with salt and pepper.

3. Place the flour in a bowl, and dig the chicken in the flour until it is softly covered.

4. Heat the oil in an enormous skillet over medium-high warmth.

5. Add the chicken to the skillet and dark-colored on the two sides, 3-4 minutes for each side.

6. When the chicken is done, expel it from the dish and put it in a safe spot.

7. Turn the warmth down to medium. Add the spread and mushrooms to a similar dish and sauté until the mushrooms are delicate (around 5 minutes).

8. When the mushrooms are done, including the wine or chicken soup to deglaze the dish and mix well.

9. Add the chicken back to the container and cook until sauce has thickened (around 2 minutes).

Dietary data (per serving):

289 calories, 9 g carbs, 18 g fat, 26 g protein, 329 mg sodium

Marinated mushroom sandwich

In this formula, mushrooms are the stars rather than meat on the grounds that the final product is lower in fat, making this sandwich simpler to process. For individuals with reflux disease, this is significant in light of the fact that nourishment with a great deal of fat can draw out stomach acid emission and exacerbate reflux disease symptoms. Olive oil is utilized rather than margarine or different fats like mayonnaise since it contains fundamental solid fats with no soaked fat. The feta cheddar is solid in season, so it gives the fulfillment of cheddar, yet very little is required. Blending the cheddar in with basil and olive oil makes an artificial pesto aioli with fewer calories and fat at that point if mayonnaise had been utilized, further bringing down the general fat substance. There is additionally a great deal of fiber in this formula, which is a sustenance suggestion for those with reflux disease.

Formula serves 4

Entire wheat pasta serving of mixed greens

This formula gives heaps of fiber and sound fats to keep you full. It likewise has numerous nutrients and minerals from the entire grains, sound herbs, and crisp vegetables. It has a Greek flare and is made with entire wheat pasta… and still tastes great!

The vast majority of us consider pasta plate of mixed greens, and we consider loads of mayonnaise. In this way, here is a formula for a light summer pasta plate of mixed greens that is solid and tastes extraordinary. It replaces the mayo with vinaigrette and utilizations herbs and feta cheddar to upgrade the flavor. This formula calls for cherry tomatoes. They are less acidic and somewhat better than customary tomatoes and are regularly endured by individuals with reflux disease; be that as it may, it they trouble you, have a go at supplanting them with red grapes.

Formula serves 10 (1 cup for every serving)

Asparagus quiche

This extraordinary tasting, solid quiche tops you off with protein rather than fat!

Who doesn't adore going out to breakfast and requesting the solid veggie quiche? Be that as it may, who knew what you are eating really is brimming with cream margarine and cheddar? That is a great deal of dairy and a ton of disappointment later. We made this extraordinary formula for an incredible tasting sound quiche that tops you off with protein rather than fat. It tastes and seems as though you put a ton of work into it, however, it's actually very basic.

We did a couple of things that make this conventional formula more advantageous. Turkey bacon replaces customary bacon to diminish the fat. Swiss and Parmesan cheeses are utilized, which are loaded with enhancing, enabling you to utilize less and decrease the general fat substance of the formula, yet at the same time get the fulfillment of cheddar. Be that as it may, the principal offender in this dish is cream; creamer, which is the most minimal fat cream, still contains 18% fat! Supplanting the cream it with plain, nonfat yogurt makes the equivalent rich surface, however, is such a great amount of better for your wellbeing.

Formula serves 8

Ingredients:

- ❖ 1 unbaked, 9-inch piecrust
- ❖ ½ pound asparagus cut into ¼ inch pieces (or somewhere in the range of 1 and 1 ½ cups)
- ❖ 6 turkey bacon strips, cooked to wanted freshness and slashed
- ❖ ½ C Swiss cheddar
- ❖ ¼ C Parmesan cheddar
- ❖ ½ tbsp. salt
- ❖ 1/8 tbsp. nutmeg

Bearings:

1. Preheat the stove to 450^0, spread piecrust with aluminum thwart and heat for 5 minutes, evacuate the foil, and prepare for 5 extra minutes.

2. Steam asparagus until brilliant green and delicate, yet at the same time fresh (around 4-5 minutes).

3. While cooking the asparagus, beat the eggs in a bowl and gradually include the yogurt ½ cup at once.

4. Add in the nutmeg, salt, chives, and mix.

5. Slowly include the cheeses, leaving a modest quantity to sprinkle on the highest point of the quiche.

6. Once the bacon is cooked, add to the egg blend.

7. When the piecrust is done, and the asparagus has been steamed, spread the asparagus over the base of the piecrust.

8. Slowly pour the egg-yogurt blend over the highest point of the asparagus; this will give the last item a layered look.

9. Spray the rest of the cheddar.

10. Reduce the broiler temperature to 400^0 and prepare the quiche in for 10 minutes; at that point, diminish the warmth 350^0 and keep heating for 25-30 minutes. The quiche is done when a blade is embedded in the focal point of the quiche and tell the truth.

11. Let stand 15-20 minutes before serving. This guarantees the quiche won't self-destruct.

Nourishing data (per serving):

200 Calories, 11 g fat, 16 g starch, 3 g fiber, 15 g protein, 83 mg cholesterol, 338 mg sodium

Banana Ginger Energy Smoothie

Ingredients

- ❖ ½ cup ice
- ❖ 2 cups of milk
- ❖ 2 bananas, ready
- ❖ 1 cup yogurt
- ❖ ½ tbsp. crisp ginger, stripped and ground fine
- ❖ 2 tbsp. dark-colored sugar or nectar (discretionary)

Headings

1. In a blender, including the ice, milk, yogurt, bananas, and ginger.

2. Mix until smooth.

3. Include sugar varying.

Function Apple Honeydew Smoothie

Ingredients

- ❖ 2 cups honeydew melon (stripped, seeded, cut into lumps)
- ❖ 4 tbsp. crisp aloe vera, skin expelled
- ❖ 1 Gala apple (stripped, cored, cut down the middle)
- ❖ 1/16 tbsp. lime pizzazz (utilize a grater to get the get-up-and-go)
- ❖ 1 ½ cups ice
- ❖ ¼ tbsp. salt

Headings

1. In a blender, including the melon, ice, aloe vera, apple, salt, and lime pizzazz.

2. Start mixing on Pulse before changing to High. Stop and mix the blend varying to get a smooth consistency.

Muesli-Style Oatmeal

Ingredients

- ❖ 1 cup moment oatmeal
- ❖ 1 cup milk
- ❖ 2 tbsp. raisins (heated to the point of boiling, depleted)
- ❖ ½ banana, diced
- ❖ ½ brilliant apple, stripped, diced
- ❖ Spot of salt
- ❖ 2 tbsp. sugar or nectar

Headings

1. The prior night (or if nothing else 2 hours prior), blend the oatmeal, milk, raisins, salt, and sugar (or nectar) together in a bowl.

2. Spread and spot in the cooler.

3. Include natural product before serving.

4. If the blend is excessively thick, including milk.

Moment Polenta With Sesame Seeds

Ingredients

- ❖ ¾ cup moment polenta or cornmeal
- ❖ 3 cups entire milk
- ❖ 3 tbsp. dark-colored sugar
- ❖ 1 tbsp. orange concentrate
- ❖ ½ tbsp. vanilla concentrate
- ❖ Salt to taste
- ❖ 1 tbsp. sesame seeds

Bearings

1. Heat the milk.

2. Include the polenta or cornmeal and whisk energetically to forestall knots.

3. Cook until rich.

4. Include the sugar, salt, and vanilla, and orange concentrate just before serving.

Quiet Carrot Salad

Ingredients

- ❖ 1 lb. carrots (stripped, cut, and ground)
- ❖ ¼ lb. mesclun greens
- ❖ 2 tbsp. raisins
- ❖ 2 tbsp. squeezed orange
- ❖ 1 tbsp. dried oregano
- ❖ 2 tbsp. dark-colored sugar
- ❖ 2 tbsp. olive oil
- ❖ ¼ tbsp. salt

Bearings

1. In a bowl, blend the raisins, squeezed orange, oregano, dark colored sugar, olive oil, and salt. Let sit for around 5 minutes.

2. Pour the dressing over the carrots and blend all together.

3. Season with extra salt, varying.

4. Serve over mesclun leaves.

Dark Bean and Cilantro Soup

Ingredients

- ❖ 8 oz. canned dark beans
- ❖ 1 16 ounces chicken stock
- ❖ ½ cup new cilantro
- ❖ Salt to taste
- ❖ 1 tbsp. nonfat harsh cream

Headings

1. Heat the chicken stock to the point of boiling. Include the beans, cilantro, and salt.

2. Cook 30 minutes on low warmth.

3. Mix with a hand blender to the ideal consistency.

4. Season, varying.

5. Serve in a soup bowl and topping with 1 tbsp.: nonfat acrid cream and a sprig of cilantro.

Cooked fish and appreciate!

Formula serves four

Chicken and Mushroom Cheese Bake

With fall rapidly drawing closer, our considerations pattern away from the grill, and we begin to consider "comfort foods." This prepared goulash formula is one of our family's top choices. It utilizes low-fat ingredients like skim milk and diminished fat cheddar to make it heartburn inviting. Include a solid portion of steamed broccoli for an ideal side dish. Tasty Cantaloupe Gazpacho

<u>Ingredients</u>

1 lb. (2 cups) melon (skin expelled, seeded, cut into 1-inch pieces)

- ❖ 2 tbsp. dark-colored sugar or agave sugar
- ❖ 2 tbsp. port wine
- ❖ Cleaning of fine-ground nutmeg

Bearings

1. Blend the melon, sugar, and port — the spot in the cooler for around 4 hours.

2. Mix in a blender.

3. Finish with the cleaning of nutmeg.

4. Serve promptly in a shot glass or little cup.

Rich Hummus

Ingredients

- ❖ 1 can (19 oz.) canned chickpeas (depleted and washed twice)
- ❖ 1 cup chicken stock
- ❖ 2 tbsp. olive oil
- ❖ ¼ tbsp. sesame oil
- ❖ ½ tbsp. salt

Bearings

1. Spot the chickpeas in a nourishment processor and include the chicken stock, olive oil, sesame oil, and salt.

2. Procedure until smooth.

3. Include chicken stock varying.

4. Serve cold with toast focuses, stove toasted corn chips, or little wedges of flatbread.

Watermelon and Ginger Granite

Ingredients

- ❖ 3 cups seedless watermelon juice (mixed)
- ❖ 1 cup of water
- ❖ ½ cup nectar
- ❖ 1 entire clove
- ❖ 1 squeeze ground nutmeg
- ❖ 1 tbsp. new ginger
- ❖ 1 tbsp. salt
- ❖ ½ tbsp. lemon get-up-and-go

Asparagus quiche

This incredible tasting, sound quiche tops you off with protein rather than fat!

Who doesn't cherish going out to breakfast and requesting the sound veggie quiche? Yet, who knew what you are eating really is brimming with cream margarine and cheddar? That is a ton of dairy and a great deal of disappointment later. We made this extraordinary formula for an incredible tasting sound quiche that tops you off with protein rather than fat. It tastes and seems as though you put a great deal of work into it, yet it's actually very basic.

We did a couple of things that make this conventional formula more advantageous. Turkey bacon replaces ordinary bacon to lessen the fat. Swiss and Parmesan cheeses are utilized, which are loaded with enhancing, enabling you to utilize less and diminish the general fat substance of the formula, yet at the same time get the fulfillment of cheddar. However, the fundamental guilty party in this dish is cream; creamer, which is the least fat cream, still contains 18% fat! Supplanting the cream it with plain, nonfat yogurt makes the equivalent velvety surface, yet is such a great amount of better for your wellbeing.

Formula serves 8

Ingredients:

- ❖ 1 unbaked, 9-inch piecrust
- ❖ ½ pound asparagus cut into ¼ inch pieces (or somewhere in the range of 1 and 1 ½ cups)
- ❖ 6 turkey bacon strips, cooked to wanted freshness and hacked
- ❖ 2 green onion or chives
- ❖ 5 eggs (or 2 eggs and 3 egg whites/1 egg and 3 egg whites)
- ❖ 1.5 C nonfat or low-fat plain yogurt (Greek yogurt can be utilized yet might be progressively tart in enhancing)
- ❖ ½ C Swiss cheddar
- ❖ ¼ C Parmesan cheddar

- ❖ ½ tbsp. salt
- ❖ 1/8 tbsp. nutmeg

Directions:

1. Preheat the broiler to 450⁰, spread piecrust with aluminum thwart and prepare for 5 minutes, expel the foil, and heat for 5 extra minutes.

2. Steam asparagus until brilliant green and delicate, yet at the same time fresh (roughly 4-5 minutes).

3. While cooking, beat the eggs in a bowl and gradually include the yogurt ½ cup at once.

4. Add in the nutmeg, salt, chives, and mix.

5. Slowly include the cheeses, leaving a limited quantity to sprinkle on the highest point of the quiche.

6. Once the bacon is cooked, add to the egg blend.

7. When the piecrust is done, and the asparagus has been steamed, spread the asparagus over the base of the piecrust.

8. Slowly pour the egg-yogurt blend over the highest point of the asparagus; this will give the last item a layered look.

10. Reduce the broiler temperature to 400^0 and prepare the quiche in for 10 minutes. At that point, lessen the warmth 350^0 and keep heating for 25-30 minutes. The quiche is done when a blade is embedded in the focal point of the quiche and tell the truth.

11. Let stand 15-20 minutes before serving. This guarantees the quiche won't self-destruct.

Banana Ginger Energy Smoothie

Ingredients

- ❖ ½ cup ice
- ❖ 2 cups of milk
- ❖ 2 bananas, ready
- ❖ 1 cup yogurt
- ❖ ½ tbsp. crisp ginger, stripped and ground fine
- ❖ 2 tbsp. dark-colored sugar or nectar (discretionary)

Directions

1. In a blender, including the ice, milk, yogurt, bananas, and ginger.

2. Mix until smooth.

3. Include sugar varying.

Function Apple Honeydew Smoothie

Ingredients

- ❖ 2 cups honeydew melon (stripped, seeded, cut into lumps)
- ❖ 4 tbsp. crisp aloe vera, skin expelled
- ❖ 1 Gala apple (stripped, cored, cut down the middle)
- ❖ 1/16 tbsp. lime pizzazz (utilize a grater to get the get-up-and-go)
- ❖ 1 ½ cups ice
- ❖ ¼ tbsp. salt

Directions

1. In a blender, including the melon, ice, aloe vera, apple, salt, and lime pizzazz.

2. Start mixing on Pulse before changing to High. Stop and mix the blend varying to get a smooth consistency.

Muesli-Style Oatmeal

Ingredients

- ❖ 1 cup moment oatmeal
- ❖ 1 cup milk
- ❖ 2 tbsp. raisins (heated to the point of boiling, depleted)
- ❖ ½ banana, diced
- ❖ ½ brilliant apple, stripped, diced
- ❖ Spot of salt
- ❖ 2 tbsp. sugar or nectar

Directions

1. The prior night (or if nothing else 2 hours prior), blend the oatmeal, milk, raisins, salt, and sugar (or nectar) together in a bowl.

2. Spread and spot in the fridge.

3. Include natural product before serving.

4. I the blend is excessively thick, including milk.

Moment Polenta with Sesame Seeds

Ingredients

- ❖ ¾ cup moment polenta or cornmeal
- ❖ 3 cups entire milk
- ❖ 3 tbsp. darker sugar
- ❖ 1 tbsp. orange concentrate
- ❖ ½ tbsp. vanilla concentrate
- ❖ Salt to taste
- ❖ 1 tbsp. sesame seeds

Directions

1. Warm the milk to boiling.

2. Include the polenta or cornmeal and whisk overwhelmingly to forestall protuberances.

3. Cook until rich.

4. Include the sugar, salt, and vanilla, and orange concentrate just before serving.

Quiet Carrot Salad

Ingredients

- ❖ 1 lb. carrots (stripped, cut, and ground)
- ❖ ¼ lb. mesclun greens
- ❖ 2 tbsp. raisins
- ❖ 2 tbsp. squeezed orange
- ❖ 1 tbsp. dried oregano
- ❖ 2 tbsp. dark-colored sugar
- ❖ 2 tbsp. olive oil
- ❖ ¼ tbsp. salt

Directions

1. In a bowl, blend the raisins, squeezed orange, oregano, dark colored sugar, olive oil, and salt. Let sit for around 5 minutes.

2. Pour the dressing over the carrots and blend all together.

3. Season with extra salt, varying.

4. Serve over mesclun leaves.

Dark Bean and Cilantro Soup

Ingredients

- ❖ 8 oz. canned dark beans
- ❖ 1 16 ounces chicken stock
- ❖ ½ cup new cilantro
- ❖ Salt to taste
- ❖ 1 tbsp. nonfat acrid cream

Directions

1. Heat the chicken stock to the point of boiling. Include the beans, cilantro, and salt.

2. Cook 30 minutes on low warmth.

3. Mix with a hand blender to the ideal consistency.

4. Season, varying.

5. Serve in a soup bowl and embellishment with 1 tbsp.: nonfat acrid cream and a sprig of cilantro.

Delightful Cantaloupe Gazpacho

Ingredients

- ❖ 1 lb. (2 cups) melon (skin evacuated, seeded, cut into 1-inch pieces)
- ❖ 2 tbsp. dark-colored sugar or agave sugar
- ❖ 2 tbsp. port wine
- ❖ Cleaning of fine-ground nutmeg

Directions

1. Blend the melon, sugar, and port — a spot in the cooler for around 4 hours.

2. Mix in a blender.

3. Finish with the cleaning of nutmeg.

4. Serve promptly in a shot glass or little cup.

Rich Hummus

Ingredients

- ❖ 1 can (19 oz.) canned chickpeas (depleted and washed twice)
- ❖ 1 cup chicken stock
- ❖ 2 tbsp. olive oil
- ❖ ¼ tbsp. sesame oil
- ❖ ½ tbsp. salt

Directions

1. Spot the chickpeas in a nourishment processor and include the chicken stock, olive oil, sesame oil, and salt.

2. Procedure until smooth.

3. Include chicken stock varying.

4. Serve cold with toast focuses, broiler toasted corn chips, or little wedges of flatbread.

Watermelon and Ginger Granite

Ingredients

- ❖ 3 cups seedless watermelon juice (mixed)
- ❖ 1 cup of water
- ❖ ½ cup nectar
- ❖ 1 entire clove
- ❖ 1 squeeze ground nutmeg
- ❖ 1 tbsp. new ginger
- ❖ 1 tbsp. salt
- ❖ ½ tbsp. lemon get-up-and-go

Butternut squash soup

In the event that you love investing energy with loved ones during the Christmas season, one of your fundamental past occasions during this season is eating. This formula is an incredible tasting first course that is warm, filling, stuffed with nutrients and minerals, and, obviously, delectable – ideal for a virus winter night!

The formula sounds somewhat extraordinary – practically startling – in case you're not used to utilizing various flavors, however, the flavors meet up superbly. As far back as I thought of the formula, I am continually approached to cause it for each event I to visit. The yellow curry powder isn't spicy. However, it is an incredible flavor enhancer, and nutmeg is a mystery fixing in a considerable lot of my plans.

It is low in calorie, brimming with nutrients K, A, C, all the B nutrients, magnesium, potassium, cancer prevention agents, and fiber. It is likewise incredible for your financial limit!

Formula serves 8-10

Broiler steamed tilapia

This formula is flavorful, solid, and quick to make – ideal for a bustling weeknight!

A few people with reflux disease avoid fish dishes since they are regularly matched with citrus – lemon and lime – which can make their reflux symptoms erupt. Be that as it may, this formula is really stomach-settling because of the ginger.

It matches pleasantly with an Asian vegetable, like bokchoy or sautéed snow peas, and dark colored rice. Keep in mind, however, that rice takes significantly longer to cook than this dish, so prepare. Whatever it is presented with, steaming the fish in material paper cooks it flawlessly.

Mustard pork midsection with cauliflower puree

This formula is somewhat unique since I truly needed to feature the side dish, yet in addition, give you something to go with it. I have been making this a great deal recently in light of the fact that, obviously, my new year's resolution is to eat superior to a year ago. My principle accentuation is devouring more vegetables, and I need to consider imaginative thoughts, so I don't get exhausted with them!

The cauliflower in this formula is an incredible, sound swap for a starch; it has surface and tops you off like pureed potatoes. However, it is a lot of lower in calories. It tastes extraordinary, as well. The pork flank is a low fat cut of pork and, for the most part, has less immersed fat than red meat. This is an incredible dish if your husband is a fundamentals type, or you need to fool your children into eating vegetables. This is likewise an extraordinary turn on comfort nourishment for a cool day.

Formula serves 4

Stuffed mushroom tops

I generally have a stomachache for around three days after the game from my non-GERD well-disposed nourishment decisions. So here is an appetizing formula that you can bring to a gathering, realizing that your companions won't think you are insane for attempting to bring something sound. And it's not veggies and plunge – as a rule, the default "sound thing" on the smorgasbord table. You can even now be unique, get your Vitamins D, An, E, and a considerable lot of the B's AND keep your GERD under control. You can make this veggie lover by forgetting about the turkey bacon. However, bacon is constantly a group pleaser, particularly when football is included!

Formula Serves 6-10 (you can twofold or triple formula varying)

Ingredients:

- ❖ 2 cloves Garlic
- ❖ ½ cup Breadcrumbs
- ❖ 6 Slices Turkey Bacon, cooked firm and disintegrated
- ❖ 5 oz Spinach hacked
- ❖ ¼ C Gruyere – ground
- ❖ ¼ C Romano – ground
- ❖ 24 medium estimated mushrooms, white or dark-colored stems expelled (Save the stems to cleave and blend in with different ingredients)
- ❖ ¼ C Olive oil

Directions:

1. Preheat stove to 375^0.

2. Bake mushroom tops on a lubed treat sheet top looking up for around 10 minutes.

3. Chop garlic, mushroom stems, and turkey bacon. Saute in olive oil over medium warmth until all are delicate and starting to darker (around 5 minutes).

4. Add spinach and keep sautéing for 3 minutes more until spinach is withered.

5. In an enormous bowl blend, breadcrumbs, and cheddar. When the stove blend is done, add it to the bowl with breadcrumbs and cheddar. Consolidate completely.

6. Fill the mushroom tops with the blend.

7. Place on the prepared sheet a subsequent time and heat again for 10-15 additional minutes.

Dietary data (per serving):

Calories 105, Fat 7g, Carbohydrates 6g, Fiber 1g, Protein 5g, Cholesterol 60mg, Sodium 800mg.

Braised short ribs

Tumble off-the-bone ribs. Sounds tasty, isn't that right? This exemplary dish is ideal for the moderate cooker on a virus winter day. And combined with bunches of veggies, this dish sneaks up all of a sudden.

However, the jumps in the lager give it a decent flavor. The liquor vanishes in the cooking procedure, so it shouldn't influence your GERD symptoms. The stock is stacked with nutrients and minerals from cooking the bones, herbs, and veggies. One other thing to note – it's prescribed to restrain red meat when you have GERD in view of the high-fat substance. This formula, as readied, just has 9 grams of fat for every serving on the grounds that the fat cooks off as you braise the ribs and winds up in the fluid. Make certain to utilize an opened spoon when serving this dish to leave the fat in the pot.

I combined this with my prior formula for cauliflower puree, and they taste extraordinary together! Spot the meat and veggies directly over the puree to make them pop.

The dish rushes to assemble, yet it takes a couple of hours to slow cook. You can simply leave it on the burner or in the moderate cooker while you clean the house for your visitors… possibly. Appreciate!

Formula serves 4

Little lasagna cups

It's the ideal opportunity for some franticness! If you are going to any ball watch gatherings or plan to have your own, this dish is quick, simple to make, and a positive group pleaser.

To begin with, this formula utilizes basil pesto rather than tomato sauce. You can make your own pesto, however, after all the ongoing occasion meals and with Easter right around the bend, I am going to make it straightforward, and we will purchase the sauce. To lessen the aggregate sum of fat and increment the measure of protein in this dish, we'll use curds rather than ricotta and ground turkey rather than a ground hamburger. The pesto sauce contains fat. However, it is sound fat, and pesto is brimming with nutrients and minerals from the herbs, just as calcium and nutrient D from the cheddar.

If you are a veggie-lover, take a stab at subbing sautéed, cleaved mushrooms for the ground turkey.

Formula serves 12

Ingredients:

- ❖ 6 oz. (around 1/3 pound) ground turkey
- ❖ 1 cup low or non–fat curds
- ❖ 1 ½ cups part-skim mozzarella cheddar
- ❖ 1 ½ cups destroyed parmesan cheddar
- ❖ 1 cup pesto sauce (basil and parsley mix)
- ❖ 24 wonton wrappers

Directions:

1. Preheat broiler to 375⁰.

2. Prepare a biscuit tin by showering every one of the 12 openings with a canola or olive oil splash.

3. Brown the ground turkey in a skillet. Add salt and pepper to taste.

4. Place a wonton wrapper in every biscuit cup and push down into the biscuit cups.

5. In each cup, layer the three kinds of cheese, at that point, the meat, at that point, pesto.

6. Place another wonton wrapper on top and continue layering.

7. Top with the rest of the mozzarella and parmesan cheddar.

8. Bake for 15-20 minutes until the cheddar is dissolved, and the wonton wrappers are sautéed.

9. Carefully expel from biscuit tin and cool before serving.

10. A basil leaf or Kalamata olive (with pit evacuated) makes a decent topping!

Dietary data (per serving):

Calories 197, Fat 12g, Carbohydrates 11g, Fiber 2g, Protein 11g, Cholesterol 13mg, Sodium 400mg

Smaller than usual lasagna cups

It's the ideal opportunity for some franticness! On the off chance that you are going to any ball watch gatherings or plan to have your own, this dish is quick, simple to make, and a clear group pleaser.

Initially, this formula utilizes basil pesto rather than tomato sauce. You can make your own pesto, however, after all the ongoing occasion meals and with Easter right around the bend, I am going to make it basic, and we will purchase the sauce. To lessen the aggregate sum of fat and increment the measure of protein in this dish, we'll use curds rather than ricotta and ground turkey rather than ground meat. The pesto sauce contains fat. However, it is solid fat, and pesto is brimming with nutrients and minerals from the herbs, just as calcium and nutrient D from the cheddar.

If you are a veggie-lover, take a stab at subbing sautéed, hacked mushrooms for the ground turkey.

Formula serves 12

Ingredients:

- ❖ 6 oz. (around 1/3 pound) ground turkey
- ❖ 1 cup low or non–fat curds
- ❖ 1 ½ cups part-skim mozzarella cheddar
- ❖ 1 ½ cups destroyed parmesan cheddar
- ❖ 1 cup pesto sauce (basil and parsley mix)
- ❖ 24 wonton wrappers

Directions:

1. Preheat broiler to 375⁰.

2. Prepare a biscuit tin by showering every one of the 12 openings with a canola or olive oil splash.

3. Brown the ground turkey in a skillet. Add salt and pepper to taste.

4. Place a wonton wrapper in every biscuit cup and push down into the biscuit cups.

5. In each cup, layer the three kinds of cheese, at that point, the meat, at that point, pesto.

6. Place another wonton wrapper on top and continue layering.

7. Top with the rest of the mozzarella and parmesan cheddar.

8. Bake for 15-20 minutes until the cheddar is softened, and the wonton wrappers are cooked.

9. Carefully expel from biscuit tin and cool before serving.

10. A basil leaf or Kalamata olive (with pit evacuated) makes a decent embellishment!

Dietary data (per serving):

Calories 197, Fat 12g, Carbohydrates 11g, Fiber 2g, Protein 11g, Cholesterol 13mg, Sodium 400mg

Formula serves 10

Handcrafted granola parfait

This flexible formula has everything: protein, fiber, solid fats, and heaps of nutrients and minerals. Attempt it today for breakfast or a sound bite!

This formula is incredible for a fast, sound breakfast since it's stacked with nourishment: fiber from the oats, protein from the Greek yogurt, solid fats from the almonds, and nutrients and minerals from the natural product. It is additionally impeccable to bring to an early lunch and can make a pleasant blessing. I like to make a major bunch of this granola, place it in sacks, and tie some strip around the pack with a tag with the dietary data to give as a blessing to my associates. Adorable, solid, and scrumptious!

Plans serve 16 (1/4 cup for every serving)

Enchiladas Verde

This interpretation of conventional Mexican nourishment is helped up and adjusted for individuals with acid reflux, so you can appreciate the kind of Mexican nourishment without the torment.

I LOVE Mexican nourishment. However, I as a rule lament eating it on the grounds that the tomatoes and flavors regularly leave me with heartburn. Rather than a customary red sauce, this formula utilizes a Verde or green; sauce produced using tomatillos. It's light on the warmth, yet at the same time gives the wonderful taste of Mexican nourishment without the agony later. Obviously, everyone has various triggers, so you ought to avoid tomatillos on the off chance that you discover they are a trigger for you.

I likewise made a couple of different changes to settle on this a solid decision for individuals with GERD. I utilized yogurt rather than acrid cream to lessen the measure of fat in the dish in light of the fact that numerous Mexican dishes will, in general, be high in fat, which can intensify symptoms of GERD. I utilized chicken thighs in this formula, yet you could utilize chicken bosoms in the event that you needed to decrease the fat substance much more – simply know that the bosoms will, in general, be on the drier side.

These enchiladas are additionally stuffed with sustenance. I utilized corn tortillas, which are a lot higher in fiber than flour tortillas. The herbs and vegetables utilized in the sauce are high in nutrients C and K, there is calcium in the cheddar and yogurt, and garlic is stuffed with cell reinforcements. And the capsaicin in the peppers has mitigating properties. On the off chance that you like some flavor, keep the seeds in the peppers. If you don't care for it by any stretch of the imagination, expel them. Remember, the yogurt added to the sauce will lessen the warmth, also.

Formula serves 8 (2 enchiladas for each serving)

Pasta primavera with entire wheat pasta

Alfredo sauce for individuals with GERD? It sounds insane. However, this adjustment of the customary family recipe provides the entirety of the flavor without the entirety of the fat, so you can appreciate this dish without paying for it later.

I am certain when you read this formula title; you were likely frightened. Alfredo sauce is famously high in fat, yet it is one of my preferred foods! I have a formula that my grandma gave me, yet it calls for overwhelming whipping cream in the sauce, and I end up with repulsive heartburn and stomach torment each time I make it. I modified this family formula, so I can, at present, appreciate it and make something my grandma made, yet with a solid wind. I trust you appreciate it, as well!

I helped up the sauce to make it simpler to process since high-fat foods can be an issue for individuals with heartburn. Despite the fact that this is a lighter adaptation of a customary dish. It additionally has numerous B nutrients and iron from the entire grains, calcium from the milk and spread substitute, Vitamin D in the mushrooms and dairy, and the asparagus is high in the two nutrients K and A.

Formula serves 8

Curry almond chicken

This is a decent, light summer dish. I, for the most part, pair this with dim green veggies, and since the curry gives the chicken a yellow shading, it makes a fun, brilliant plate. Curry is regularly a misjudged flavoring. Numerous gentle curries can include a lot of flavor to a dish without bothering GERD as spicy flavors can. What's more, curry powder is made with turmeric, which contains an incredible cell reinforcement. Curiously, some examination proposes that turmeric has hostile to disease properties that could be valuable to GERD patients who are increasingly vulnerable to Barrett's Esophagus.

This formula is stuffed with protein from the chicken and almond milk, yet expelling the skin from the chicken keeps the fat substance low. And the almond milk includes a solid portion of calcium. Appreciate!

Formula serves 6

Balsamic Chicken Salad

This balsamic chicken plate of mixed greens is a meal in itself. Great balsamic vinegar is produced using grapes, and there are numerous impostors out there, so make certain to check the fixing name, and search for the words "matured grapes must" or "Mostod'Uva." The matured vinegar has a dim shading and a somewhat sweet and rich flavor that loans itself well to an assortment of vinaigrette dressings and gourmet sauces – and it gives the perfect punch to this GERD-accommodating dish. We include hacked apples, crisp greens, lentils, celery, parsley, and ginger to finish the dish. It's one of a kind, sound, and rich enough for organization!

Makes 4 servings

Ingredients

- ❖ 3 TBSP.P. Olive Oil
- ❖ 4 skinless, boneless chicken bosom (4 oz.)

- ❖ 1/2 tbsp. ginger
- ❖ 1/4 tbsp. pepper
- ❖ 1/4 tbsp. salt
- ❖ 2 TBSP.P.Balsamic vinegar
- ❖ 2 stalks celery, daintily cut
- ❖ 1 Green Apple, cleaved
- ❖ 2 TBSP.P. Apple Juice
- ❖ 1 15-oz can new lentils, washed
- ❖ 2 cups new greens, hacked
- ❖ 1/2 cup cleaved new parsley

Directions

1. Season chicken with ginger and pepper

2. Heat the olive oil and Include chicken bosoms and cook until brilliant dark colored around 8 to 10 minutes for every side

3. Remove from warmth and coat well with vinegar

4. In an enormous plate of mixed greens bowl, hurl the celery, hacked apple and squeezed apple, staying 2 TBSP.P.olive oil and salt

5. Fold in the crisp greens, lentils, and parsley and present with chicken

Wholesome ingredients per serving:

Calories 165, Sat fat .9 g, Sodium 575 mg.

1 tbsp. of Balsamic vinegar contains 2.4 grams of sugar so, on the off chance that you are diabetic, you may be cautious about the amount you devour

Cooked salmon with mango nectar soy coat

This formula is anything but difficult to get ready and so scrumptious even the individuals who are not huge salmon fans will adore it.

The sound advantages incorporate mango, which is wealthy in dietary fiber, and nectar, which can assist work with increasing vulnerabilities (since nearby nectar has dust from your territory). Salt and pepper and garlic are discretionary. For the individuals who can endure scallions, put a couple of cuts over the

Formula serves 4-6

Chicken tortilla soup

Nothing hits the spot like a warm, healthy soup on a crisp fall evening. Decreased fat tortilla chips give a pleasant surface to our sound formula of chicken tortilla soup. Top your bowl with low fat destroyed Monterey Jack or cheddar. Prepare a fresh ice shelf lettuce plate of mixed greens to balance a delectable meal!

Formula serves 4

Coconut rice pudding

Coconuts contain regular sugar and can be a heavenly and sound approach to add some sweetness to your diet. There are no "trigger" ingredients in this formula, and we have seen visit exchange on the Internet about coconut being useful to GERD sufferers – you should be the judge! This formula is speedy and simple and wind on an unsurpassed, most loved pastry. However, for those viewing their cholesterol, remember that coconut milk contains some soaked fat, so this formula probably won't be the correct decision for you.

Makes around 6 servings

Ingredients

- ❖ 3/4 cup low-fat milk
- ❖ 1/2 cup coconut milk
- ❖ 1 enormous pear ground
- ❖ 2 tbsp..nectar
- ❖ 1 (1oz) bundle moment fat-free, sugar-free vanilla pudding blend

- ❖ 2 cups cooked rice
- ❖ 1/4 cup destroyed coconut
- ❖ 1/2 tbsp. ground ginger

Directions

Heat the initial four recorded ingredients to the point of boiling over medium warmth and quickly expel from heat. Gradually blend in the pudding with a wire whisk. Mix in rice, coconut, and ginger. Let blend sit for 10 minutes to mix favors, mixing once in a while. Top with berries whenever wanted. It can be served warm or cold.

Dietary data (per serving):

190 Calories, 6 g fat, 31 g sugar, 3 g protein, 2 mg cholesterol, 244 sodium

Sweet pea smoothie

Peas have never tasted so sweet! I have a smoothie each morning, and I like to switch back and forth between 100% natural product smoothies and foods grown from the ground smoothies. This sound formula of peas, pineapple, banana, and strawberry makes a special and delicious smoothie, and it is one of my top picks! It is ideal for an early in the day bite, and it delightfully sneaks an extra part of vegetables into your GERD diet. An early in the day tidbit can assist you with eating increasingly visit, littler meals during the day to assist you with dealing with your bit size, a key for individuals with GERD. Simply join the ingredients in the blender, mix until smooth, and voila! We're almost certain you won't be ravenous for a major lunch!

Formula serves 2

Ingredients

- ❖ 1/2 cup pineapple juice
- ❖ 1 cup solidified strawberries
- ❖ 1/3 cup solidified peas
- ❖ 1 banana

Directions

1. Cook peas as per bundle directions, at that point flush, channel, and cool.

2. Place the cooked peas in the blender

3. Add the rest of the ingredients, spread, and mix on fast until smooth (around 30 seconds)

4. Pour the blend into two glasses and appreciate it!

Wholesome data (per serving):

190 calories, calories from fat 0, all out starch 43g (dietary fiber 5g, sugars 26g), cholesterol 0, Sodium 25mg, complete fat 1/2 g, protein 3g

Chicken and Red Potatoes

With beautiful olives and carrots, this appealing chicken and fresh red potato dish are staggering for organization and helpful enough for occupied weeknights as well. It's anything but difficult to season and set up the red potatoes and carrots in the broiler, mix once and add them to a meal dish with the remainder of the ingredients, including chicken, green olives, dried rosemary, and tart apple juice. Chicken and red potatoes are a GERD-accommodating formula and a general sound across the board meal. Present with asparagus and a serving of mixed greens or rice as an afterthought, and you'll have a total and satisfying menu. Appreciate!

Makes four serve

Ingredients

❖ 12 oz red potatoes, cut into one inch solid shapes

- ❖ 2 enormous carrots, stripped and cut into 1-inch pieces
- ❖ 2 TBSP.P.olive oil
- ❖ 1/4 tbsp. genuine salt
- ❖ 1/4 tbsp. turmeric
- ❖ 2 cups pre-cooked chicken meat, destroyed or cleaved
- ❖ 1/2 tbsp. dried rosemary
- ❖ 1/3 cup pitted green olives
- ❖ 2 TBSP.P.apple juice (or squeezed apple)
- ❖ 2 TBSP.P.crisp parsley (discretionary)

Directions

1. Preheat broiler to 425

2. Tossed potatoes, carrots together with oil, salt, and turmeric

3. Spread uniformly onto a rimmed heating sheet

4. Bake until delicate around 35 minutes, blending once halfway

5. Transfer to a goulash dish, mix in chicken, rosemary, olives and squeezed apple

6. Cook for 10 additional minutes until warmed through

7. Serve quickly, hurled with parsley whenever wanted

Nourishing ingredients per serving:

Calories 335, Sat fat 2.4, Sodium 258 mg.

Simple hamburger (or pork) burgundy

There are times when no one but meat can fulfill your taste buds, and this great dish works for me! Since meat is harder to process than different foods, we recommend that you utilize just a lean hamburger, limit the recurrence of meat in your meals, and keep the bit size little. For this formula, we suggest that you use hamburger tenderloin, a less fatty cut of meat. For an intriguing turn and a lower fat variant, pursue similar directions yet substitute a similar size pork tenderloin for the hamburger tenderloin! Make sure to restrain the meat part to a sound 3.5 oz and top off on the veggies. And don't stress over the red wine – the liquor will dissipate during cooking.

Serves 4

Stuffed turkey moves "cordon bleu."

This stuffed and moved dish is amusing to make, so put on your innovative cap and check out it. It requires a little exertion, yet we promise it merits the time. We overlooked salt and did a light sprinkle of pepper on every cutlet, and increase the flavor by blending thyme and ginger into the bread pieces. These two flavors are considered the GERD diet inviting, so appreciate!

Makes 4 servings

Ingredients

- ❖ 4 – 1/4 pound turkey bosom cutlets
- ❖ 1/2 teaspoon dark pepper
- ❖ 4 (1ounce) cuts smoked ham, low fat, low sodium
- ❖ 2 (1 ounce) decreased fat Swiss cheddar cuts
- ❖ 3 Tablespoons plain dry bread pieces
- ❖ 1 teaspoon dried thyme
- ❖ 1/2 teaspoon ground ginger
- ❖ 1 Tablespoon low-fat mayonnaise

- ❖ 1/4 cup dry white wine
- ❖ 1/4 low sodium chicken soup
- ❖ 1 Tablespoon delicate margarine

Directions

1. Season the cutlets with pepper and spot 1 cut of ham and 1/2 cup of cheddar over each bit of the turkey. Move up and verify with toothpicks.

2. Mix the bread pieces with ginger and thyme.

3. Brush the moved up cutlets with the mayonnaise and coat with the breadcrumb blend. Pack them delicately, so they follow.

4. Spray an enormous skillet with nonstick cooking shower, and bring to medium warmth. Include the rolls and cook until brilliant dark colored on all sides, around 4 to 5 minutes.

5. Add the wine, margarine, and chicken stock and heat to the point of boiling. Spread the container and decrease warmth to a stew.

6. Cook around five minutes longer until the turkey is altogether cooked and the sauce thickens

Dietary data (for 1 turkey roll):

145 calories, 9 g fat, 3 g sat fat, 430 mg sodium, 5 g carbs 16 g protein.

Crisp vegetable and white bean soup

One of my preferred recollections as a child experiencing childhood in the Midwest was helping my grandmother make soup. This formula is a sound, low-sodium, low-fat adaptation of granny's soup, made with "no sodium" chicken stock and a tad of normal vegetable bouillon. What makes the soup scrumptious is the blend of crisp vegetables stewed together with the white beans. You can likewise include some destroyed cooked chicken (or ham) to the completed soup for a total meal. At that point, stir up the fire and appreciate it!

Makes four 3/4 cup servings

Prepared chicken and wild rice

There are some low-fat adaptations of chicken and rice, and we especially like this one since we utilize the flavors tarragon and ginger blended in with white wine to please add the required flavor to the sodium-free chicken broth*. We avoid additional fat in this formula by delicately poaching the chicken and vegetables in the stock before preparing it in the broiler. Both white and wild rice are incorporated, and liberal segments of cut crisp mushrooms and hacked celery complete the dish. This isn't just an ideal meal for those with acid reflux, yet it is additionally extraordinary for family meals and little social affairs. Appreciate!

Formula serves 4

Vegetable macaroni and cheddar

Macaroni and cheddar, the great 1950s solace nourishment, has made a major rebound at eateries around the nation. When finding for the most part in burger joints, "Macintosh and cheddar" has advanced into high-end foundations and is present even prominently combined with (for goodness' sake!) lobster. Despite the fact that we use vegetables rather than lobster in our GERD-accommodating variant, you can positively have some steamed lobster as an afterthought! This formula utilizes entire wheat macaroni blended in with hacked cauliflower (or celery), egg whites, and scrumptious low-fat sharp cheddar. Impeccable as a principle course or side dish, there's nothing more needed than minutes to get ready.

Makes 4 one-cup servings

Small spinach serving of mixed greens

Every one of the specialists nowadays appears to concur that eating fish is useful for your wellbeing. This serving of mixed greens formula is GERD cordial and one of our top choices, and it's an innovative method to add some additional fish to your diet. The blend of shrimp, strawberries, and asparagus is consummately combined with a raspberry vinaigrette and beat for mash with fragmented almonds. The dish is low in calories, yet filling, so it makes an extraordinary lunch or light supper. Even better, we figure it may even fulfill your sweet tooth as well!

Makes four servings

Barbecued Caesar swordfish

Swordfish is a mainstream and solid fish. It is low in calories, however high in protein, and has a consistency that makes it flawless the barbecue! For this formula, we first marinate the fish in a diminished fat Caesar plate of mixed greens dressing for 30 minutes. This gives the fish an interesting flavor that sets pleasantly with the romaine lettuce leaves. These ingredients are low in fat and GERD diet agreeable, yet on the off chance that you can endure a sprinkle of lemon, take the plunge! Present with flame-broiled vegetables hurled with a scramble of balsamic vinegar to balance the meal.

Makes six servings

Lentil burgers

You may be wondering why, lentils? To begin with, lentils are heavenly and flexible enough to make a delicious and solid adaptation of a "cheeseburger." Second, lentils are a plant protein that will give your body supplements, for example, molybdenum, folate, and manganese, which are huge supporters of heart wellbeing. Third, lentils are filling, yet low in calories and contain essentially no fat. And to wrap things up, lentils are GERD benevolent and don't advance heartburn! This formula additionally contains cleaved kale*, ground carrots, and cumin, a GERD well-disposed flavor. Serve alone or on an entire wheat bun with a chunk of ice lettuce and nectar mustard.

Serves 4

Ingredients

- ❖ 2 cups cooked lentils
- ❖ 1/2 cup dried bread morsels

- ❖ 1/2 cup egg blenders
- ❖ 1/4 cup ground carrot
- ❖ 3/4 cup slashed kale*
- ❖ 1 or 2 TBSP.P.slashed dried onion (as indicated by inclination)
- ❖ 1/4 teaspoon fit salt
- ❖ 1/2 teaspoon pepper
- ❖ 1/2 teaspoon cumin
- ❖ 1/3 cup ground sharp cheddar
- ❖ Ice shelf lettuce
- ❖ Nectar mustard dressing
- ❖ Entire wheat cheeseburger buns (toasted)
- ❖ 1 TBSP.P. Canola or olive oil

Directions

1. Combine together the cooked lentils, bread morsels, egg blenders (or two egg whites), and cheddar with the slashed kale, carrots, and fried onion. Include the flavors and structure into four 3/4 inch patties. Try not to include the oil. Chill burgers well for at any rate 1 hour on a wax paper-lined heating sheet.

2. When prepared to cook, empty the oil into a nonstick skillet and warmth until bubbly. Include the chilled burgers and decrease warmth to medium. Set a clock for 2 1/2 minutes. Flip over when the clock goes off and keep on cooking for an extra 2 to 3 minutes or until the burgers look seared and are steaming hot!

3. Lightly channel the patties on paper towels, and then serve on toasted buns with ice shelf lettuce and nectar mustard dressing.

*Fresh slashed spinach can be filled in for cleaved kale

Wholesome data (per burger):

252 calories; 5.6 g fat; 1.5 s fat; 394 g sodium; 17 g protein

Hawaiian-style ahi sandwich with coconut slaw

Need a sample of the tropics on a virus winter day? Let your taste buds transport you to Hawaii with our acid reflux-accommodating fish sandwich. Ahi fish, likewise called yellowfin, is one of the biggest of the fish species. Truth be told, one of the records gets of yellowfin fish was estimated at an incredible 300 pounds. However, in spite of its circumference, yellowfin fish is shockingly low in fat. It is likewise an incredible wellspring of a few supplements you require for good wellbeing, including protein, potassium, phosphorous, and nutrients D and B 12. These plans are simple and amusing to get ready, and we figure you will appreciate the island flavors.

Serves 2

Chicken pot pie

Chicken pot pie is a heavenly treat, yet it very well may be difficult to legitimize the calories. So we concocted this delicious, "irreproachable" adaptation of the great solace dish that makes an ideal dinner whenever – yet particularly on a stormy winter night! The formula is low calorie and GERD amicable, yet at the same time healthy and scrumptious with poached chicken, blended veggies, and a flaky pie outside.

Makes 6 to 8 servings

Ingredients

- ❖ 1 cup fat-free chicken soup
- ❖ 1 cup fat-free cream
- ❖ 3 T generally useful flour
- ❖ 1 tbsp. poultry flavoring
- ❖ 1 tbsp. thyme
- ❖ 2 cups poached white chicken meat
- ❖ I sack solidified blended vegetables (10 oz)
- ❖ 1 T dried minced onions (discretionary)

- ❖ 1 tbsp. legitimate salt
- ❖ 1/4 tbsp. pepper
- ❖ 1 instant diminished fat pie outside

Directions

1. Thaw solidified veggies and channel well (should be possible daily ahead).

2. Gently poach 2 boneless chicken bosoms in delicately salted water for around 15 minutes or until done. Try not to bubble or overcook. Cut the meat into shapes. The chicken can be readied a day ahead and kept in the cooler until prepared to utilize, or you can utilize extra chicken. can be utilized)

3. In a medium pot, combine creamer, flour, thyme, chicken juices, and poultry flavoring.

4. Bring the blend to a bubble while whisking admirably, and then diminish warmth to a stew.

5. Continue whisking the blend for another 3 to 5 minutes until it thickens.

6. Remove the dish from the warmth and mix in the cubed chicken, defrosted veggies, minced onion, and salt and pepper.

7. Place the blend into a 9-inch pie plate and top with the pie outside.

8. Cook in a preheated 425-degree stove for 30 minutes or until bubbly.

Healthful data per serving: Calories 216, Fat 4 grams

Banana date mousse

This sound mousse will securely and definitely fulfill your sweet tooth! It is an ideal light sweet formula, and it's brisk and simple to plan in your blender. We prescribe utilizing ready bananas and Medjool dates, which are non-acidic fruits that are simple on the stomach and GERD agreeable. I you have never attempted dates, they are a genuine treat and one of my preferred characteristic sugars. Like bananas, dates contain heaps of nutrients and minerals that advance great wellbeing. We utilize crude sugar in this formula. However, you may incline toward a sugar substitute.

Serves 4

Salmon burgers with carrot slaw and miso yogurt

If you like crab cakes, you will appreciate these salmon burgers since they are similarly as scrumptious and have a comparative flaky surface. This is Asian-enlivened acid reflux amicable formula is made with crisp ginger and white miso, which are both considered GERD diet neighborly flavors. For those inexperienced with white miso, it's a customary Japanese flavoring, in glue structure, produced using matured soybeans. We blend the white miso glue with plain yogurt to make a delectable low-fat, mayonnaise-style besting for the burger. A tbsp. or two of our own carrot slaw completes the sandwich, so we prescribe a durable and softly toasted cheeseburger style bun.

Serves 4

Ingredients

- ❖ 2 carrots ground
- ❖ 1 celery stalk finely chopped**
- ❖ 1 enormous egg
- ❖ 2 teaspoons rice vinegar
- ❖ 1 teaspoon canola oil
- ❖ 1/4 pound skinless salmon filet
- ❖ 1 tablespoon finely ground crisp ginger
- ❖ 1 tablespoon dried minced onion (discretionary)
- ❖ 1/2 cup Panko bread morsels
- ❖ 1/4 cup plain yogurt
- ❖ 1 teaspoon white miso*
- ❖ 4 entire wheat burger buns
- ❖ Ocean or legitimate salt and pepper

Directions

1. Add the carrots, celery, vinegar and oil in a little bowl, and put in a safe spot.

2. Cut the skinless salmon filet into 1-inch pieces.

3. In a different bowl, tenderly "hand blend" the salmon pieces, new ginger, bread morsels, enormous egg, 1/4 t pepper, and discretionary dried minced onion until the blend is consolidated.

4. Form the blend into four 3/4 inch patties and then make a little space with your thumb into the highest point of every patty. This will help avert over-plumping during cooking.

5. Cover the patties and chill in the fridge for 30 minutes to 60 minutes.

6. Lightly oil a spotless barbecue and cook the patties on medium-high for 8 to 10 minutes, delicately flipping once at the midpoint until patties look obscure. Toast the buns on the barbecue.

7. Place the cooked patties onto the readied buns and top each with a tablespoon or a greater amount of miso yogurt (formula pursues) and the ideal measure of carrot slaw.

Miso Yogurt

Blend 1/4 cup plain yogurt with 1 teaspoon white miso* (soybean glue) until consolidated.

Dietary data (per serving):

410 calories, 619 mg sodium, 11 g fat, 127 mg cholesterol

Smooth split pea soup

Split peas are GERD agreeable and pressed with sound nutrients and supplements, including potassium, fiber, and protein. This soup is heavenly and ideal for a crisp night, and it's likewise an incredible method to utilize an extra ham bone. We utilize low sodium chicken soup in this formula and flavor it up with heaps of heartburn amicable seasonings. A liberal measure of carrots and celery with a scramble of discretionary dried onions complete the dish. Be certain not to hold back on the cooking time in light of the fact that the peas taste best when they arrive at a "velvety" consistency. Appreciate!

Makes around 6 servings

Ingredients

- ❖ 1 ham bone
- ❖ 1 pound split peas
- ❖ 8 cups low sodium chicken stock

- ❖ 1 cup cleaved celery
- ❖ 2 to 3 diced carrots
- ❖ 1 Tablespoon dried cleaved onion*
- ❖ 1 narrows leaf
- ❖ 1/2 teaspoon thyme
- ❖ 1/2 teaspoon ginger
- ❖ 1/2 teaspoon pepper
- ❖ 1/2 teaspoon marjoram
- ❖ 1/4 teaspoon dried mustard

<u>Directions</u>

1. Rinse peas well and assess and take out all flotsam and jetsam.

2. In a huge stockpot, heat chicken juices to the point of boiling.

3. Add ham bone and stew for 45 minutes.

4. Remove ham bone and permit to cool.

5. Add cleaned peas, all seasonings, and remaining ingredients to the dish, and come back to a bubble. Lessen warmth to a low stew and spread the dish. Stew

on low for at any rate one hour or until the peas nearly break down.

6. Stir regularly to avoid consuming, and if the soup gets excessively thick, include more stock.

7. When prepared to serve, take the meat out the ham bone and come back to the pot, mix well, and spoon into soup bowls.

*dried slashed onions are more GERD cordial than new onions, yet avoid them on the off chance that they trigger your symptoms

Wholesome data (per serving):

Calories 266, Sat fat 4.5 grams, Sodium 369 grams.

Great morning natural product plate of mixed greens

A natural product plate of mixed greens is a decent and solid approach to begin your day. This formula is made with GERD-accommodating fruits, including kiwi, which adds tropical energy to the dish. Kiwifruits are plentiful in fiber and contain as a lot of nutrient C as an orange, an organic citrus product a great many people with acid reflux avoid. While choosing kiwifruits, ensure they yield tenderly to pressure and avoid those that are delicate or wounded. The cutting and stripping for this blend will require a little exertion. However, it will last in any event a couple of days in the cooler.

Sound jumble plate of mixed greens

No opportunity to cook? Investigate your washroom and cooler to perceive what you have on hand that is solid and additionally GERD agreeable. We found canned fish, white beans, pecans, and dark-colored rice in the washroom, and in the ice chest, we had feta cheddar, new beets, lettuce, carrots, and a hard bubbled egg. While this is certifiably not a customary formula, a "mess" meal like this is fun, so be imaginative! It works with a heap of ingredients including cabbage, kale, arugula, mushrooms, quinoa, celery, avocado – whatever you have promptly accessible. You can likewise include remaining chicken, steak, or fish. Simply set up every one of the ingredients together in an enormous bowl, prepare with your preferred low-fat plate of mixed greens dressing, and voila! It's all set in only minutes!

Makes around 2 servings

Carrot milkshake smoothie

This smoothie formula is an ideal fast and solid breakfast for an "in a hurry" morning. On the off chance that you like carrot cake, you will appreciate the milkshake surface of this smoothie, and the mix of carrots, milk, banana, and cinnamon make it mmm flavorful! This heartburn well-disposed treat is additionally an incredible method to fulfill your sweet tooth whenever of the day while including some additional products of the soil to your acid reflux neighborly diet.

Raisin walnut and carrot bread

This delectable bread formula is low in immersed fat and is made with carrots, raisins, and walnuts, all acid reflux amicable ingredients. We utilize a modest quantity of egg in the formula. However an egg substitute will likewise function admirably for the individuals who need to limit eggs in their GERD diet plan. I make this frequently in light of the fact that my family cherishes it! It's simple, sound, and so pleasant!

The formula makes one portion (Serving size 1/2 inch cut)

Exquisite Dover sole

Dover sole is a mellow white fish with a sensitive rich flavor. It is additionally a "level" firm fish, which makes it perfect for stuffing and rolling. This formula is made with spinach and mushrooms and prepared with oregano to give it a Mediterranean pizazz. We utilize only a sparse measure of oil, and part-skim mozzarella cheddar to keep the dish low in fat and GERD diet well disposed. A scramble of garlic powder is discretionary and ought to be excluded if the dried herb triggers your heartburn symptoms.

Makes 4 servings (serving size: 1 filet roll)

Peachy shoemaker

This pastry formula demonstrates you don't need to spend too much on calories to fulfill your sweet tooth. It's made with heartburn inviting fruits and squeezes and seasoned up with nutmeg and cinnamon, which are additionally GERD diet benevolent flavors.

Makes 8 servings

Ingredients

- ❖ 1/2 tbsp. ground cinnamon
- ❖ 1 Tbsp.p. vanilla concentrate
- ❖ 2 Tbsp.p. cornstarch
- ❖ 1 cup peach nectar
- ❖ 1/4 cup pineapple squeeze or peach juice
- ❖ 2 16-oz jars peaches, cut, stuffed in juice, depleted (or 1-3/4 lbs new)
- ❖ 1 Tbsp.p. margarine
- ❖ 1 cup dry flapjack blend
- ❖ 2/3 cup generally useful flour
- ❖ 1/2 cup sugar
- ❖ 2/3 cup dissipated skim milk

- ❖ Nonstick cooking oil shower (for preparing dish)
- ❖ Beating: 1/2 tbsp. nutmeg and 1 TBSP.P.dark colored sugar

Directions

1. Add cinnamon, vanilla, cornstarch, peach nectar, and pineapple or peach squeeze in a pan over medium warmth. Mix continually until blend thickens and bubbles.

2. Add cut peaches to blend.

3. Reduce warmth and stew for 5 to 10 minutes.

4. In another pan, soften margarine and put in a safe spot.

5. Lightly shower an 8-inch square glass dish with cooking oil splash. Empty hot peach blend into the dish.

6. In another bowl, join hotcake blend, flour, sugar, and liquefied margarine. Mix in milk.

7. Quickly spoon this blend over peach blend.

8. Combine nutmeg and darker sugar. Sprinkle blend over hitter.

9. Bake at 410° F for 10 to 15 minutes or until brilliant dark-colored.

10. Cool and cut into 8 squares.

Dietary data (per serving):

Calories 271, Fat 4 g, Saturated fat under 1 g, Cholesterol under 1mg, Sodium 263 mg

Makes 18 1/2 cup servings

Outing potato serving of mixed greens

Nothing is more fundamental for a mid-year cookout than a scrumptious potato plate of mixed greens. This "All-American" crisp vegetable dish is mayo-based and prepared with flavorful flavors to give it a great deal of pizzazz. Yukon gold, fingerling, or red delight potatoes will work best for this formula since they keep their shape well when cooked. Be certain not to overcook the potatoes and to expel them from heat while still somewhat firm. We additionally prescribe flavoring the potatoes while still warm with the goal that they better ingest the flavors. It's low in fat, GERD diet inviting, and basically divine!

Makes 10 1/2-cup servings

Excursion potato plate of mixed greens

Nothing is more basic for a late spring cookout than a delightful potato plate of mixed greens. This "All-American" crisp vegetable dish is mayo-based and prepared with appetizing flavors to give it a great deal of pizzazz. Yukon gold, fingerling, or red ecstasy potatoes will work best for this formula since they keep their shape well when cooked. Be certain not to overcook the potatoes and to expel them from heat while still marginally firm. We likewise suggest flavoring the potatoes while still warm with the goal that they better assimilate the flavors. It's low in fat, GERD diet agreeable, and essentially heavenly!

Makes 10 1/2-cup servings

Meat and mushroom skillet

There are times when just a hamburger will fulfill your taste buds, and this healthy skillet formula will work! We utilized a lean cut of meat (top round) and plain low-fat yogurt to keep the dish low in fat and GERD diet inviting. We seasoned the sauce with nutmeg, ginger, and dried basil – all heartburn neighborly flavors. Make certain to restrain your hamburger part to a 3.5 oz. serving and make the most of your preferred vegetables or some dried up bread as an afterthought.

Yield: 5 servings–Serving Size: 6 oz

Ingredients

- ❖ 1 pound lean hamburger (top round)
- ❖ 3 TBSP.P.apple juice vinegar
- ❖ 2 tbsp. vegetable oil
- ❖ 3/4 TBSP.P.dried minced onion*
- ❖ 1 pound cut mushrooms
- ❖ 1/4 tbsp. salt

- ❖ Pepper to taste
- ❖ 1/4 tbsp. nutmeg
- ❖ 1/4 tbsp. ginger
- ❖ 1/2 tbsp. dried basil
- ❖ 1/4 C white wine
- ❖ 1 C plain low-fat yogurt
- ❖ 6 C cooked macaroni, cooked in unsalted water

Directions

1. Cut hamburger into 1-inch solid shapes, and marinate for in any event 2 hours in vinegar.

2. Heat 1 tbsp. oil in a non-stick skillet.

3. Add hamburger and sauté for 5 minutes. Go to dark-colored uniformly. Expel from the dish and keep hot.

4. Add residual oil to container; sauté mushrooms.

5. Add hamburger to the skillet with seasonings.

6. Add wine, yogurt, and dried onion; delicately mix in. Warmth, yet don't bubble.

7. Serve with entire wheat pasta or dark-colored rice

Note:

If thickening is wanted, utilize 2 teaspoons cornstarch; calories are equivalent to flour. However, it has a twofold thickening force. These calories are not considered along with the supplements per serving.

Healthful Information (per serving):

Calories: 499, Total fat: 10 g, Saturated fat: 3 g Cholesterol: 79 mg, Sodium: 200 mg

*Omit onions if the dried structure triggers your GERD symptoms

Prepared French fries

Who doesn't cherish French fries? However, fries without ketchup? We, as a whole, realize that tomato-based ketchup can trigger GERD symptoms, so we prepare these fries in this formula to extra fresh, which makes them impeccable to dunk in apple juice vinegar. If you have never attempted fries dunked in vinegar, you are in for a treat. Stove preparing makes these potatoes lower in fat than their fried cousins, which keeps this formula GERD diet amicable. And recollect, fries are best when they are fresh outwardly and velvety within, so don't half-cook!

Makes 5 servings–Serving size: 1 cup

Ingredients

- ❖ 4 enormous Russets or Idaho potatoes (2 lbs)
- ❖ 8 cups of ice water
- ❖ Apple juice vinegar
- ❖ 1 tbsp. garlic powder*
- ❖ 1 tbsp. onion powder*

- ❖ 1/4 tbsp. salt
- ❖ 1 tbsp. white pepper
- ❖ 1/4 tbsp. allspice
- ❖ 1 Tbsp.p. vegetable oil

Directions

1. G the potatoes and cut them into long 1/2-inch strips.

2. Place potato strips into ice water, spread, and chill for 1 hour or more.

3. Remove potatoes and dry strips altogether.

5. Toss potatoes in flavor blend.

6. Brush potatoes with oil.

7. Place potatoes in nonstick shallow preparing skillet.

8. Cover with aluminum foil and spot in 475° F stove for 15 minutes.

9. Remove foil and keep heating revealed for an extra 15 to 20 minutes or until brilliant dark colored and firm!

10. Turn fries once in a while too dark-colored on all sides.

Nourishing data (per serving):

Calories 238, Fat 4 g, Saturated fat 1 g, Cholesterol 0 mg, Sodium 163 mg

*If the dried type of these herbs trigger your GERD symptoms, preclude or substitute with your most loved GERD amicable flavor.

Outlandish Asian rice

This formula utilizes an assortment of ingredients, including walnuts and water chestnuts, to make this an interesting side dish for any meal. Additionally utilize a modest quantity of a new onion, yet whenever cooked onion triggers your heartburn symptoms, substitute it with an identical measure of dried onion, or exclude them from the formula. Green pepper, celery, and long grain rice, prepared with sage and nutmeg complete the dish! Mmm, you will enjoy the outlandish flavor!

The formula makes 10 1/2 cup servings.

Home-style southern bread rolls

Bread rolls have, for some time, been a staple of the American diet, particularly in Southern states. Crisply prepared promptly in the first part of the day, breakfast rolls are a convention in the South and eaten with nectar, margarine, syrup, or jams. They additionally make an ideal backup for supper soups and stews. We helped up the good old form to make them GERD diet amicable, so you all appreciate it! This formula is finger-licking' great!

Makes 15 2-inch bread rolls

Heated bananas

This basic formula is delectable and a superb treat for breakfast or pastry. Bananas are normally sweet, wealthy in solid potassium, and are viewed as a sheltered organic product for individuals who have acid reflux. Different ingredients, including coconut, ginger, and cinnamon, are GERD diet cordial. For breakfast, I serve the bananas alone or with oatmeal as an afterthought – or beat with hacked nuts or raisins in the event that I have them on hand. For an after supper treat, I appreciate them with a scoop of solidified yogurt! Mmm great!

Serves 6

Twice heated potatoes

This vegetable dish is scrumptious and made with GERD diet amicable ingredients, including the flavors dill and ginger. The potatoes are twice heated and then stuffed, which requires some additional time – yet you will believe it merits the exertion! It's an ideal side dish for an evening gathering and matches well with meat, fish, or fowl. The formula is low fat, low-cholesterol, and low-sodium treat, and can be made a day ahead for ease.

Makes 8 servings (1/2 potato for every serving)

Frosty mango smoothie

Mangoes taste so great that individuals may overlook that they are additionally sound, containing high measures of fiber, iron, and cell reinforcements. Its organic product enhance is frequently depicted as a fascinating blend of pineapple and peach. Sounds heavenly! And what's more, they are GERD diet well-disposed and don't advance heartburn symptoms. Grown-ups and children the same will cherish the smooth sweet taste of this beverage! It's an ideal breakfast for your GERD diet design or whenever of the day as a meal substitution.

Makes 4 servings (3/4 cup for each serving)

Carolina potato pie

This "low nation" roused sweet potato pie is helped up to make it GERD diet benevolent. We utilize vegetable oil (rather than spread) and dissipated skim milk to work. Sweet potatoes are stacked with sound fiber, potassium, and nutrient An and have a couple of fewer calories than their white partner. This vegetable dish formula is a wonderful side for merry evening gatherings, occasions, and family meals, and matches superbly with pork, poultry, or meat.

Makes 16 servings

Apple smoothie with wheat germ

This apple smoothie with wheat germ is a GERD diet well disposed, starch-rich, mixture that makes certain to give you a stimulating lift! It makes a decent early in the day or evening nibble. Wheat germ is the most nutritious piece of the wheat grain. It's pressed with protein, minerals, and nutrients B and E, making it an excessively sound expansion to any smoothie. Empty it into your blender, include yogurt, a ready banana, squeezed apple, a tablespoon of flax seeds, and voila! This formula makes an ideal tonic for general prosperity in not more than seconds!

Makes two 6 oz. servings

Ingredients

- ❖ 2 TBSP.P.Wheatgerm
- ❖ 1 enormous ready banana
- ❖ 1/2 cup plain yogurt
- ❖ 1 TBSP.P.flax seeds
- ❖ 1 cup squeezed apple

❖ 1/4 cup water*

Directions

1. Place the wheat germ, 2/3 of the banana, yogurt, and flax seeds in a blender or nourishment processor.

2. Blend until smooth and mix well.

3. Add the squeezed apple to the blend and mix once more.

4. Pour into an enormous glass and top with water and remaining banana cuts.

Wholesome data (per serving):

Calories 179, Sat fat 1g, Sodium 58mg

*Try antacid water to support the manifestation battling capability of this smoothie.

Structure your own' breakfast granola

Granola is over the top expensive to purchase at the store, however reasonable to make at home, so put on your innovative cap and check out this formula. It's simple since granola is fundamentally simply moved oats to which you can include your decision of dried fruits, nuts, and other delicious goodies. You can likewise change the blend with GERD diet cordial flavors like cinnamon and ginger. Include the flavors and ingredients like darker sugar, ground apple, and coconut before heating. Different decisions like dried fruits, nuts, and raisins ought to be included in the wake of preparing. It's a quite sympathetic formula, so don't hesitate to have a fabulous time while tweaking your own mix!

Ingredients

- ❖ 6 cups moved oats
- ❖ 6 cups wheat germ
- ❖ 1 cup plate of mixed greens oil
- ❖ 1 cup nectar
- ❖ Also your preferred additional items like flavors, coconut, raisins, almonds, or different nuts and dried fruits

Directions

1. Mix oats and wheat germ in a huge bowl.

2. Mix oil and nectar together, at that point, add to the primary blend.

3. If you're utilizing additional ingredients like flavors, dark colored sugar, ground apple, or coconut, include them before heating.

4. Bake at 350 degrees on treat sheets for 15 minutes.

5. You may need to mix with a fork to ensure all get dry.

6. Add your additional items like raisins, almonds, different nuts, or dried foods grown from the ground.

7. Let set to cool, at that point, store in a hermetically sealed holder.

Nourishing data (per half-cup serving):

Approximately 120 calories, sat fat 2g, sodium 31. However, this is, to a great extent, reliant on what you include.

Natively constructed turkey soup

The blend of a huge assortment of flavors stewed with an extra turkey cadaver gives the juices in this well-known soup formula an extraordinary and astonishing flavor. The turkey corpse ought to have in any event two cups of meat staying on it to make a decent, rich soup. We keep the soup lower in soaked fat and GERD diet cordial by setting it up early, enabling it to cool, and then skimming off the fat that ascents to the top.

The formula makes around 16 1-cup servings

White Fish Veronica

Prepared crisp white fish, a scramble of lemon, and loads of seedless grapes join to make a luscious and sound GERD diet agreeable dish. Low-sodium chicken soup and low-fat milk lessen the fat substance for this formula, yet still give the sauce a rich, velvety taste. Pick one of the fish types recorded beneath, and utilize them.

Makes 4 servings

Vegetarian chia burger

Chia is a modest little seed with enormous nourishment, including iron, omega 3, magnesium, calcium, and selenium. Goodness! What's more, chia is known to give a full feeling, which can assist you with avoiding gorging – a key factor for an effective GERD diet. The seeds are anything but difficult to mix it up of plans, including soups, sauces, smoothies, and burgers. We joined chia seeds with sunflower seeds, slashed almonds, and coconut oil to give this veggie lover burger a wonderful "nutty" season. It's delectable, sweet, and so special!

Yields 6 servings and can without much of a stretch be multiplied to make 12

CPSIA information can be obtained
at www.ICGtesting.com
Printed in the USA
BVHW040148160721
612110BV00006B/22